Bone and Cartilage Conduction

Bone and Cartilage Conduction

Guest Editor
Tadashi Nishimura

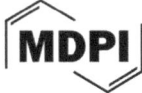

Basel • Beijing • Wuhan • Barcelona • Belgrade • Novi Sad • Cluj • Manchester

Guest Editor
Tadashi Nishimura
Otolaryngology-Head and
Neck surgery
Nara Medical University
Kashihara
Japan

Editorial Office
MDPI AG
Grosspeteranlage 5
4052 Basel, Switzerland

This is a reprint of the Special Issue, published open access by the journal *Audiology Research* (ISSN 2039-4349), freely accessible at: https://www.mdpi.com/journal/audiolres/special_issues/bone_cartilage_conduction.

For citation purposes, cite each article independently as indicated on the article page online and as indicated below:

Lastname, A.A.; Lastname, B.B. Article Title. *Journal Name* **Year**, *Volume Number*, Page Range.

ISBN 978-3-7258-3825-7 (Hbk)
ISBN 978-3-7258-3826-4 (PDF)
https://doi.org/10.3390/books978-3-7258-3826-4

© 2025 by the authors. Articles in this book are Open Access and distributed under the Creative Commons Attribution (CC BY) license. The book as a whole is distributed by MDPI under the terms and conditions of the Creative Commons Attribution-NonCommercial-NoDerivs (CC BY-NC-ND) license (https://creativecommons.org/licenses/by-nc-nd/4.0/).

Contents

Tadashi Nishimura
Bone and Cartilage Conduction
Reprinted from: *Audiol. Res.* 2022, 12, 77–78, https://doi.org/10.3390/audiolres12010007 1

Susan E. Ellsperman, Emily M. Nairn and Emily Z. Stucken
Review of Bone Conduction Hearing Devices
Reprinted from: *Audiol. Res.* 2021, 11, 207–219, https://doi.org/10.3390/audiolres11020019 . . . 3

Enrico Muzzi, Valeria Gambacorta, Ruggero Lapenna, Giulia Pizzamiglio, Sara Ghiselli, Igor Caregnato, et al.
Audiological Performance of ADHEAR Systems in Simulated Conductive Hearing Loss: A Case Series with a Review of the Existing Literature
Reprinted from: *Audiol. Res.* 2021, 11, 537–546, https://doi.org/10.3390/audiolres11040048 . . . 16

Kimio Shiraishi
Sound Localization and Lateralization by Bilateral Bone Conduction Devices, Middle Ear Implants, and Cartilage Conduction Hearing Aids
Reprinted from: *Audiol. Res.* 2021, 11, 508–523, https://doi.org/10.3390/audiolres11040046 . . . 26

Tadashi Nishimura, Tadao Okayasu, Akinori Yamashita, Hiroshi Hosoi and Tadashi Kitahara
Perception Mechanism of Bone-Conducted Ultrasound and Its Clinical Use
Reprinted from: *Audiol. Res.* 2021, 11, 244–253, https://doi.org/10.3390/audiolres11020022 . . . 42

Tadao Okayasu, Tadashi Nishimura, Akinori Yamashita, Yoshiki Nagatani, Takashi Inoue, Yuka Uratani, et al.
Word Categorization of Vowel Durational Changes in Speech-Modulated Bone-Conducted Ultrasound
Reprinted from: *Audiol. Res.* 2021, 11, 357–364, https://doi.org/10.3390/audiolres11030033 . . . 52

Tadashi Nishimura, Hiroshi Hosoi, Ryota Shimokura, Chihiro Morimoto and Tadashi Kitahara
Cartilage Conduction Hearing and Its Clinical Application
Reprinted from: *Audiol. Res.* 2021, 11, 254–262, https://doi.org/10.3390/audiolres11020023 . . . 60

Ryota Shimokura, Tadashi Nishimura and Hiroshi Hosoi
Vibrational and Acoustical Characteristics of Ear Pinna Simulators That Differ in Hardness
Reprinted from: *Audiol. Res.* 2021, 11, 327–334, https://doi.org/10.3390/audiolres11030030 . . . 69

Ronny Suwento, Dini Widiarni Widodo, Tri Juda Airlangga, Widayat Alviandi, Keisuke Watanuki, Naoko Nakanowatari, et al.
Clinical Trial for Cartilage Conduction Hearing Aid in Indonesia
Reprinted from: *Audiol. Res.* 2021, 11, 410–417, https://doi.org/10.3390/audiolres11030038 . . . 77

Sakie Akasaka, Tadashi Nishimura, Hiroshi Hosoi, Osamu Saito, Ryota Shimokura, Chihiro Morimoto and Tadashi Kitahara
Benefits of Cartilage Conduction Hearing Aids for Speech Perception in Unilateral Aural Atresia
Reprinted from: *Audiol. Res.* 2021, 11, 284–290, https://doi.org/10.3390/audiolres11020026 . . . 85

Noritaka Komune, Yoshie Higashino, Kazuha Ishikawa, Tomoko Tabuki, Shogo Masuda, Kensuke Koike, et al.
Management of Residual Hearing with Cartilage Conduction Hearing Aid after Lateral Temporal Bone Resection: Our Institutional Experience
Reprinted from: *Audiol. Res.* **2021**, *11*, 263–274, https://doi.org/10.3390/audiolres11020024 . . . **92**

Miriam Geal-Dor and Haim Sohmer
How Is the Cochlea Activated in Response to Soft Tissue Auditory Stimulation in the Occluded Ear?
Reprinted from: *Audiol. Res.* **2021**, *11*, 335–341, https://doi.org/10.3390/audiolres11030031 . . . **104**

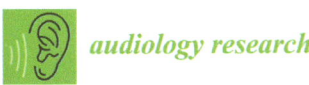

Editorial

Bone and Cartilage Conduction

Tadashi Nishimura

Department of Otolaryngology-Head & Neck Surgery, Nara Medical University, Nara 634-8521, Japan; t-nishim@naramed-u.ac.jp

Auditory sensation is an important sensation for human beings. The auricle collects sound and directs it to the auditory canal. The input sound travels to the eardrum to drive it. The vibration of the eardrum is transmitted to the cochlea via the ossicles. This is the predominantly transmission pathway to the cochlea and is termed air conduction (AC). Conversely, the sound is transmitted to the cochlea via the skull bone instead of through the AC. This pathway efficiently functions when a vibrator is placed on the bony tissue, such as the mastoid or the forehead. This pathway is termed bone conduction (BC). The details of the transmission pathways in BC are complicated. Several participating components contribute to the thresholds.

BC has usually been utilized in alternative devices for patients who are unable to use AC hearing devices or experience difficulty in benefiting from them. The progression of BC hearing devices has been slow compared to that of AC hearing devices due to the complicated pathways, problems associated with the transducer fixation, and poor demand. Recently, various hearing devices utilizing BC and implantable BC devices have been developed. Furthermore, many studies have assessed auditory sensation when transducers are placed on non-osseous tissues and have promoted its clinical use. These non-osseous types of conduction have the potential for new hearing options since the characteristics of these conductions are different from both AC and BC. The applications of these devices are still under development, and the types of conduction remain controversial. Thus, the current Special Issue focused on not only BC but also non-osseous conductions.

This issue covers topics relating to implantable BC devices, ADHEAR systems, and sound localization in BC, which is an important function in auditory sensation [1–3]. Moreover, the current issue includes bone-conducted ultrasonic perception [4,5]. Ultrasound is audible when it is presented via BC. Bone-conducted ultrasonic hearing may contribute to medical innovation since it can be perceived even in some profoundly deaf patients.

In addition to BC, the current Special Issue covers the topics of cartilage conduction (CC) and soft tissue conduction [6–11]. In particular, CC, in which the transducer is placed on the aural cartilage, is highlighted, owing to the benefits and advantages of its devices in atretic ears. CC hearing aids have already been used in clinical practice in Japan since 2017 and have gained popularity, surpassing implantable BC devices in terms of the number of new cases. These new hearing devices will be available in other countries [11], and several patients will benefit from them in the near future. This Special Issue provides up-to-date information on these novel hearing aids.

The scientific collection presented herein will hopefully be of interest to different types of professionals, such as audiologists, otolaryngologists, physiologists, and acoustical engineers.

Funding: This research received no external funding.

Institutional Review Board Statement: Not applicable.

Informed Consent Statement: Not applicable.

Data Availability Statement: Not applicable.

Citation: Nishimura, T. Bone and Cartilage Conduction. *Audiol. Res.* 2022, 12, 77–78. https://doi.org/10.3390/audiolres12010007

Received: 11 January 2022
Accepted: 14 January 2022
Published: 18 January 2022

Publisher's Note: MDPI stays neutral with regard to jurisdictional claims in published maps and institutional affiliations.

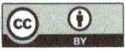

Copyright: © 2022 by the author. Licensee MDPI, Basel, Switzerland. This article is an open access article distributed under the terms and conditions of the Creative Commons Attribution (CC BY) license (https://creativecommons.org/licenses/by/4.0/).

Acknowledgments: I kindly thank all the authors for their participation and contributions to the volume, as well as all the reviewers, who have substantially contributed to the high quality of this literature. I also highly appreciate the editorial support provided by *Audiology Research*.

Conflicts of Interest: The author declares no conflict of interest.

References

1. Ellsperman, S.E.; Nairn, E.M.; Stucken, E.Z. Review of Bone Conduction Hearing Devices. *Audiol. Res.* **2021**, *11*, 207–219. [CrossRef] [PubMed]
2. Muzzi, E.; Gambacorta, V.; Lapenna, R.; Pizzamiglio, G.; Ghiselli, S.; Caregnato, I.; Marchi, R.; Ricci, G.; Orzan, E. Audiological Performance of ADHEAR Systems in Simulated Conductive Hearing Loss: A Case Series with a Review of the Existing Literature. *Audiol. Res.* **2021**, *11*, 537–546. [CrossRef] [PubMed]
3. Shiraishi, K. Sound Localization and Lateralization by Bilateral Bone Conduction Devices, Middle Ear Implants, and Cartilage Conduction Hearing Aids. *Audiol. Res.* **2021**, *11*, 508–523. [CrossRef] [PubMed]
4. Nishimura, T.; Okayasu, T.; Yamashita, A.; Hosoi, H.; Kitahara, T. Perception Mechanism of Bone-Conducted Ultrasound and Its Clinical Use. *Audiol. Res.* **2021**, *11*, 244–253. [CrossRef] [PubMed]
5. Okayasu, T.; Nishimura, T.; Yamashita, A.; Nagatani, Y.; Inoue, T.; Uratani, Y.; Yamanaka, T.; Hosoi, H.; Kitahara, T. Word Categorization of Vowel Durational Changes in Speech-Modulated Bone-Conducted Ultrasound. *Audiol. Res.* **2021**, *11*, 357–364. [CrossRef] [PubMed]
6. Nishimura, T.; Hosoi, H.; Shimokura, R.; Morimoto, C.; Kitahara, T. Cartilage Conduction Hearing and Its Clinical Application. *Audiol. Res.* **2021**, *11*, 254–262. [CrossRef] [PubMed]
7. Komune, N.; Higashino, Y.; Ishikawa, K.; Tabuki, T.; Masuda, S.; Koike, K.; Hongo, T.; Sato, K.; Uchi, R.; Miyazaki, M.; et al. Management of Residual Hearing with Cartilage Conduction Hearing Aid after Lateral Temporal Bone Resection: Our Institutional Experience. *Audiol. Res.* **2021**, *11*, 263–274. [CrossRef] [PubMed]
8. Akasaka, S.; Nishimura, T.; Hosoi, H.; Saito, O.; Shimokura, R.; Morimoto, C.; Kitahara, T. Benefits of Cartilage Conduction Hearing Aids for Speech Perception in Unilateral Aural Atresia. *Audiol. Res.* **2021**, *11*, 284–290. [CrossRef] [PubMed]
9. Shimokura, R.; Nishimura, T.; Hosoi, H. Vibrational and Acoustical Characteristics of Ear Pinna Simulators that Differ in Hardness. *Audiol. Res.* **2021**, *11*, 327–334. [CrossRef] [PubMed]
10. Geal-Dor, M.; Sohmer, H. How Is the Cochlea Activated in Response to Soft Tissue Auditory Stimulation in the Occluded Ear? *Audiol. Res.* **2021**, *11*, 335–341. [CrossRef] [PubMed]
11. Suwento, R.; Widodo, D.W.; Airlangga, T.J.; Alviandi, W.; Watanuki, K.; Nakanowatari, N.; Hosoi, H.; Nishimura, T. Clinical Trial for Cartilage Conduction Hearing Aid in Indonesia. *Audiol. Res.* **2021**, *11*, 410–417. [CrossRef] [PubMed]

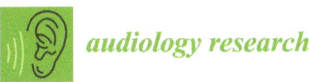 *audiology research*

Review

Review of Bone Conduction Hearing Devices

Susan E. Ellsperman *, Emily M. Nairn and Emily Z. Stucken

Department of Otolaryngology—Head and Neck Surgery, University of Michigan, Ann Arbor, MI 48109, USA; emnairn@med.umich.edu (E.M.N.); estucken@med.umich.edu (E.Z.S.)
* Correspondence: sellsper@med.umich.edu

Abstract: Bone conduction is an efficient pathway of sound transmission which can be harnessed to provide hearing amplification. Bone conduction hearing devices may be indicated when ear canal pathology precludes the use of a conventional hearing aid, as well as in cases of single-sided deafness. Several different technologies exist which transmit sound via bone conduction. Here, we will review the physiology of bone conduction, the indications for bone conduction amplification, and the specifics of currently available devices.

Keywords: bone conduction; bone-anchored hearing aid; osseointegrated implant; transcutaneous bone conduction; percutaneous bone conduction

1. Introduction

The concept of bone conduction hearing, the phenomenon through which a vibrating object can transmit sound, was first described in writing in the 1500s and credited to Girolamo Cardano [1]. Rudimentary devices such as a rod or spear were initially utilized as assistive devices for those with hearing loss by providing a route for vibrations to reach the listener. As technology advanced and the carbon microphone was developed in the early 1900s, bone conduction devices designed to convert sounds into mechanical signals that vibrate the mastoid bone were created. Early devices were held in place with a headband or eyeglasses and proved to be beneficial despite the cumbersome design and inefficient sound transmission. These early investigations paved the way for the development of modern bone-anchored hearing aids surgically implanted into the temporal bone. In 1977, Anders Tjellström and his colleagues in Sweden were the first to implant a percutaneous titanium device utilizing an osseointegrated screw [2]. The concept of osseointegration, direct contact between living osteocytes and the titanium implant, was developed by Brånemark and initially utilized for dental implants [3]. The first bone-anchored hearing device became widely commercially available in the 1980s, and since that time, patients with conductive hearing loss (CHL), mixed hearing loss (MHL), and unilateral hearing loss or single-sided deafness (SSD) have benefitted from these devices [4]. This review aims to provide an overview of bone conduction hearing physiology and the currently available bone conduction hearing devices including the indications, fitting range, benefits, and drawbacks of each.

2. Bone Conduction Physiology

Multiple physiologic mechanisms contribute to bone conduction hearing. Put simply, sound energy is transmitted from vibrations in the skull to the cochlea, which ultimately results in wave propagation along the basilar membrane and stimulation of the cochlear nerve—the same endpoint as air conduction hearing [5]. There is ongoing investigation to fully describe the mechanisms by which bone conduction hearing occurs and the relative contributions of each pathway. Five major pathways were well summarized by Stenfelt and Goode in 2005 [6]. In their review of previously published data and their own findings, they describe (1) sound radiation to the external ear canal, (2) middle ear ossicle inertia, (3)

Citation: Ellsperman, S.E.; Nairn, E.M.; Stucken, E.Z. Review of Bone Conduction Hearing Devices. *Audiol. Res.* **2021**, *11*, 207–219. https://doi.org/10.3390/audiolres11020019

Academic Editor: Tadashi Nishimura

Received: 12 March 2021
Accepted: 6 May 2021
Published: 18 May 2021

Publisher's Note: MDPI stays neutral with regard to jurisdictional claims in published maps and institutional affiliations.

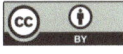

Copyright: © 2021 by the authors. Licensee MDPI, Basel, Switzerland. This article is an open access article distributed under the terms and conditions of the Creative Commons Attribution (CC BY) license (https://creativecommons.org/licenses/by/4.0/).

inertia of cochlear fluids, (4) compression of the cochlear walls (or inner ear compression), and (5) pressure transmission from cerebrospinal fluid (CSF) as the principal contributors to bone conduction. Inertia of cochlear fluids is felt to be the most important contributor [6].

Bone conduction hearing aids take advantage of the above mechanisms by converting sound energy into skull vibrations. Since the initial work by Tjellström [2] and his colleagues, there have been numerous commercial devices introduced, including surgically implanted and extrinsically applied devices. These devices are intended to assist with hearing rehabilitation for patients with conductive or mixed hearing loss who are unable to utilize conventional air conduction hearing aids or for patients with single-sided deafness. The ability to use conventional, transcanal devices may be limited by recurrent infections such as chronic otitis externa, prior surgical intervention and altered anatomy, microtia or anotia, canal atresia or stenosis, or other anatomic constraints. In the single-sided deafness population, bone conduction devices route signals transcranially to the contralateral, normal hearing cochlea.

When choosing a bone conduction device, many factors must be considered. Each patient has unique needs which are related to their degree and type of hearing impairment, anatomy, vocational or educational needs, and personal preferences. Finding this information in a consolidated location can be challenging for patients and providers. The goal of this review is to provide an overview of the current device landscape including the hearing losses best treated by each device, surgical and nonsurgical advantages and disadvantages for each class of devices, magnetic resonance imaging (MRI) compatibility, processor characteristics, wireless connectivity, and available accessories. The following description of devices includes products currently available and utilized in the United States. While meant to be inclusive of all manufacturers and products, devices in the ever-evolving landscape may have been inadvertently excluded or developed following the preparation of this review.

3. Currently Available Devices

3.1. Surgically Implanted Devices

Surgically implanted bone conduction devices convert acoustic sound waves into mechanical vibration, which is conducted to the inner ear via direct contact with the skull. These can be classified broadly into percutaneous and transcutaneous devices based on the presence or absence of a skin-penetrating abutment. The transcutaneous devices can be further classified into active and passive implants. Passive transcutaneous devices have an implanted portion of the device in direct connection with the skull and a separate, external portion held in place magnetically which drives vibration through the skin to the implanted device. In a passive system, vibration occurs at the level of the external processor, and vibrations are transmitted transcutaneously to the implanted device. Active transcutaneous devices contain an external microphone and processor which send electronic signals to an implanted, vibrating device in direct contact with the skull. With an active system, the external processor is static and transmits electronic signals. Vibration occurs at the level of the implanted device only. Currently available devices including indications for the selection of each, benefits, and drawbacks will be discussed.

3.1.1. Percutaneous Devices

Direct contact with the skull affords a meaningful advantage for percutaneous devices over passive transcutaneous devices. Passive transcutaneous devices rely on vibratory signal delivery through the skin and are subject to signal attenuation up to 20 dB, especially at high frequencies [7]. The direct connection of the percutaneous devices allows for efficient signal transmission at all frequencies without skin and soft tissue impedance. Surgical insertion of percutaneous devices is performed under local or general anesthesia through a variety of skin incisions [8]. Single-stage procedures are now standardly utilized except in situations with concern for poor wound healing or poor bone mineralization in which a two-stage operation may be considered. Traditionally, the sound processor is activated and loaded onto the abutment three months post-operatively, but the recent literature has examined the role for earlier activation at one to two weeks, or even one day post-operatively without sacrificing implant stability [9–11].

The most significant disadvantage of percutaneous implants is the potential for adverse skin reactions, device extrusion, and the need for revision surgery. The reported complication rate varies widely and appears to be influenced by the surgical technique, surgeon experience, patient age, and patient factors predisposing to infection or poor wound healing. Surgery for the placement of a percutaneous abutment was often performed with skin grafting in the past; however, skin grafting is no longer performed regularly which has resulted in overall improved cosmesis with fewer graft complications. Adverse skin reactions continue to be the most common complication of percutaneous devices, and can be categorized using the Holgers classification, a scale from zero to four described in Table 1 [12]. A 2016 systematic review published by Mohamad et al. included 30 published studies and cites a skin complication rate ranging from 9.4 to 84% [13]. A 2013 meta-analysis by Kiringoda and Lustig included 2310 implants and cited a rate of grade 2 or higher skin complications ranging from 2.4 to 38.1% [14]. The rate of revision surgery ranged from 1.7 to 34.5% in adult or mixed populations and 0 to 44.4% in pediatric populations [14].

Table 1. Holgers classification of skin complications.

Grade	Description	Management
0	No irritation	Remove epithelial debris if present
1	Slight redness	Local treatment
2	Red and slightly moist tissue (no granuloma)	Local treatment
3	Reddish and moist (may have granulation tissue)	Revision surgery indicated
4	Infection	Removal of skin penetrating implant necessary

The Holgers classification is used to classify and describe skin complications following percutaneous device placement [12].

Currently available percutaneous bone conduction devices include the Oticon Ponto System (Oticon Medical AB, Askim, Sweden) [15] and the Cochlear™ Baha® Connect System (Cochlear Bone-Anchored Solutions AB, Mölnlycke, Sweden) [16,17]. In general, these devices consist of an osseointegrated implant (screw), skin penetrating abutment, and an external sound processor. The implant and abutment may be coupled and implanted together. The devices are recommended for patients with MHL, CHL, or SSD. The degree of accepted sensorineural hearing loss varies depending on the power of the processor. In patients with a purely conductive hearing loss, those with an air–bone gap of at least 30 dB are more likely to benefit from a bone-anchored device compared to a traditional air conduction aid [18]. Patients with SSD should have a pure tone average (PTA) of better than or equal to 20 dB hearing level (HL) in the contralateral, normal hearing ear.

The Oticon Ponto became commercially available in 2009. The currently utilized implant is a 4.5-mm-wide, 6 mm long, titanium screw with an abutment [19]. Currently available processors include the Ponto 3 and Ponto 4 series devices. The Ponto 3 has three versions: Ponto 3, Ponto 3 Power, and Ponto 3 SuperPower. These processors are intended for patients with bone conduction hearing thresholds up to 45 dB HL, 55 dB HL, and 65 dB HL, respectively (Table 2; Figure 1). The Ponto 4 is a smaller device and suitable for bone conduction hearing thresholds up to 45 dB HL (Table 2; Figure 1) [15].

Table 2. Sound processor specifications.

	Device	Processor	Fitting Range	Frequency Range (DIN45.605)	Peak OFL * at 90 dB SPL	Peak OFL * at 60 dB SPL	Processing Delay	MRI Compatibility
Percutaneous	Ponto [†] [15,20]	Ponto 3	BC PTA ≤ 45 dB	200–9500 Hz	124 dB	107 dB	6 ms	Compatible up to 3 Tesla
		Ponto 3 Power	BC PTA ≤ 55 dB	260–9600 Hz	128 dB	116 dB	6 ms	
		Ponto 3 Superpower	BC PTA ≤ 65 dB	260–9600 Hz	135 dB	125 dB	6 ms	
		Ponto 4	BC PTA ≤ 45 dB	200–9500 Hz	124 dB	108 dB	8 ms	
	Baha® Connect [‡] [16,17,21,22]	Baha® 5	BC PTA ≤ 45 dB	250–7000 Hz	117 dB	105 dB	4.5 ms	Compatible up to 3 Tesla
		Baha® 5 Power	BC PTA ≤ 55 dB	250–7000 Hz	123 dB	113 dB	4.5 ms	
		Baha® 5 SuperPower	BC PTA ≤ 65 dB	250–7000 Hz	133 dB	121 dB	4.5 ms	
		Baha® 6 Max	BC PTA ≤ 55 dB	200–9700 Hz	121 dB	108 dB	<6 ms	
Transcutaneous Passive	Alpha 2 MPO [°] [23]	Alpha 2 MPO ePlus™	BC PTA ≤ 45 dB (ideal ≤ 35 dB)	125–8000 Hz	120 dB	110 dB		Compatible up to 3 Tesla
	Baha® Attract [‡] [16,17,22,24]	Baha® 5	BC PTA ≤ 45 dB	250–6300 Hz	114 dB	104 dB	4.5 ms	Compatible up to 1.5 Tesla
		Baha® 5 Power	BC PTA ≤ 55 dB	250–7000 Hz	125 dB	115 dB	4.5 ms	
		Baha® 5 SuperPower	BC PTA ≤ 65 dB	250–7000 Hz	134 dB	123 dB	4.5 ms	
		Baha® 6 Max	BC PTA ≤ 55 dB	200–9250 Hz	121 dB	108 dB	<6 ms	
Transcutaneous Active	Osia® [‡] [25–27]	Osia® 2	BC PTA ≤ 55 dB	400–7000 Hz			<6 ms	No–internal magnet must be removed
	BONEBRIDGE™ [€] [28–30]	SAMBA 2	BC PTA ≤ 45 dB	250–8000 Hz	117 dB		8 ms	Compatible up to 1.5 Tesla
Adhesive	ADHEAR [€] [31]	ADHEAR	BC PTA ≤ 25 dB	250–8000 Hz	124 dB		10 ms	Yes–remove external device

This table includes device specifics for each of the processors discussed and includes fitting ranges, frequency ranges, peak output, and MRI compatibility. (OFL = output force level relative to 1 µN on a skull simulator; * OFL may be measured at FOG (full on gain) or RTG (reference test gain), and therefore may not be directly comparable between devices). Device information is included with permission from Cochlear™, MED-EL, Medtronic, and Oticon representatives. [†] Oticon Medical AB, Askim, Sweden; [‡] Cochlear Bone-Anchored Solutions AB, Mölnlycke, Sweden; [°] Medtronic, Dublin, Ireland; MED-EL, Innsbruck, Austria; [€] MED-EL, Innsbruck, Austria.

The Cochlear™ Baha® Connect System utilizes the BI300, a titanium osseointegrated implant which is available in 3- or 4-mm lengths. The percutaneous abutment, the BA400, is hydroxyapatite-coated and is available in 6-, 8-, 10-, 12-, and 14-mm lengths to accommodate a range of soft tissue thickness [32]. The currently available series includes the Baha® 5, Baha® 5 Power, and the Baha® 5 SuperPower sound processors. These devices are intended for patients with bone conduction hearing thresholds up to 45 dB HL, 55 dB HL, and 65 dB HL, respectively (Table 2; Figure 1) [17]. To achieve a higher output, the Baha®5 SuperPower has a behind-the-ear component to allow for the physical separation of the actuator from the microphone [17]. The Baha® 6 Max was recently FDA-approved and suitable for bone conduction hearing thresholds up to 55dB HL and is anticipated to be commercially available soon (Table 2; Figure 1) [16].

The SuperPower processors for the Ponto and Baha® systems each provide powerful processors intended for patients with bone conduction hearing thresholds up to 65 dB HL. The systems have some differences that impact the fitting and use of the processors. The Ponto 3 SuperPower is one piece and less bulky than the Baha® SuperPower processor [15,17]. Feedback may be harder to control due to the inability to separate the actuator from the microphone. In contrast, the Baha® 5 SuperPower system allows for the separation of the actuator from the microphone and can be worn in several configurations for even greater separation if feedback or physical placement becomes an issue [15]. This system is larger, with two pieces, and bulkier than the Ponto 3 SuperPower device. Placement of the larger device may be challenging in patients who were initially implanted in anticipation of a standard processor but have converted to a SuperPower processor to address the worsening of sensorineural hearing. The implant placement in these patients may not be ideal to accommodate the bulkier SuperPower processor. The Baha® 5 SuperPower processor uses rechargeable batteries similar to a cochlear implant (Table 3) [17]. Available accessories and streaming capabilities are listed in Table 4.

3.1.2. Passive Transcutaneous Devices

Transcutaneous systems were designed to avoid the cosmetic concerns and skin complications associated with percutaneous devices while still delivering adequate sound transmission. In the transcutaneous systems, a titanium implant is placed directly in the skull in the same manner as the percutaneous devices. A magnet is attached to this implant, and the skin is closed over the top of the implant, avoiding a percutaneous component. Once the incision has healed and osseointegration has occurred, the external device is then activated. The external device is retained via attraction to the internal magnet and vibrates in response to sound inputs. The vibratory force then passes through the intervening skin and soft tissue to reach the internal magnet and implant which allow the transmission of the vibration to the skull.

While skin complications are less common than those seen with percutaneous devices, the magnetic force required to hold the external device in place and effectively transmit sound in transcutaneous systems can lead to pain and irritation of the intervening skin and soft tissue. When this occurs, the magnet strength can be reduced to decrease the amount of pressure applied to the skin, and users may be instructed to reduce daily wearing time or avoid using their device altogether until symptoms improve. If the amount of pressure applied is greater than the patient's capillary pressure, the skin may have inadequate blood supply and necrosis can occur [33]. A systematic review by Cooper et al. reported a 13.1% rate of minor soft tissue complications which resolved spontaneously or with use of a weaker magnet [34]. A grading system comparable to the Holgers scale for percutaneous implants has not been established; thus, reporting and comparing skin complications is challenging [12]. The rate of major complications, defined as complications requiring active management, such as post-operative seroma, hematoma, wound infections, skin ulcerations, and dehiscence, was 5.2% in the same systematic review [34].

The Baha® Attract System (Cochlear Bone-Anchored Solutions AB, Mölnlycke, Sweden) [35] and Alpha 2 MPO (formerly SOPHONO™) system (Medtronic, Dublin, Ireland) [23] are the available passive transcutaneous devices. Both devices are intended for the treatment of CHL, MHL, or SSD with normal contralateral hearing. While auditory outcomes have shown significant improvement compared to unaided conditions, signal attenuation occurs due to signal loss during transmission through the skin and soft tissues [36]. This attenuation is most apparent at high frequencies and may be as high as 25 dB at 6000 to 8000 Hz higher frequencies when compared to percutaneous devices [37,38].

The Baha® Attract uses the same BI300 implant as the percutaneous Baha® Connect. During insertion of the device, bone polishing is performed if needed to accommodate the attachment of the BIM400 implant magnet to the BI300 without the magnet making direct contact to the bone [35]. The thickness of the skin flap over the magnet must be 6mm or less, which at times may require soft tissue reduction [35]. The Baha® Attract utilizes the same external processors as the Baha® Connect intended for use with the same bone conduction hearing thresholds previously listed (Table 2; Figure 1) [16,17]. The external processors are attached to a magnet rather than directly articulating to the percutaneous post. Once adequate healing and osseointegration have taken place, the external sound processor and magnet are applied and activated. Users are instructed to begin by wearing the device a few hours a day and slowly increase usage over time to avoid skin irritation and limit discomfort. The application of a SoftWear™ pad as a barrier between the skin and device is recommended by the manufacturer [39]. Six magnets of increasing strength are available to accommodate for variable soft tissue thickness, overlying hair, and patient comfort [39]. Since the Baha® Attract and Connect devices use the universal BI300 implant, it is possible to convert from a Baha® Connect to a Baha® Attract device, though the skin at the previous abutment site must be healed and healthy prior to conversion [40,41]. The Baha® Attract is MRI compatible at 1.5 Tesla with the internal magnet in place. A sizeable area of artifact will be present on the MRI, which is significantly larger than the degree of artifact with percutaneous devices. The magnet may be surgically removed if a higher strength MRI is required or if the resultant artifact obscures critical image sequences (Table 3) [24]. Available accessories and streaming capabilities are listed in Table 4.

The Alpha 2 MPO implant system consists of two internal magnets hermetically sealed in a titanium case. This device is designed to sit within shallow bone beds which are drilled based on manufacturer recommendations. The Alpha 2 MPO device is then attached to the skull with five screws [34,37]. The Alpha 2 MPO ePlus™ sound processor is then applied and drives vibrations through the skin and soft tissue using transcutaneous energy transfer or TET™. The device is approved for patients with up to a 45 dB hearing loss with ideal candidacy up to 35 dB HL (Table 2; Figure 1) [42]. The Alpha 2 MPO system is MRI compatible up to 3 Tesla (Table 3) [28]. Available accessories and streaming capabilities are listed in Table 4.

3.1.3. Active Transcutaneous Devices

Active transcutaneous bone conduction devices were designed to maximize the benefits of percutaneous and passive transcutaneous devices while avoiding skin complications and soft tissue signal attenuation. Active devices have an external processor and implanted transducer which are connected by magnetic coils. Signals are transmitted electrically from the external to internal device using technology akin to that of cochlear implants. As the internal device is responsible for generating mechanical forces against the skull, skin attenuation does not occur, and magnet strength can be significantly reduced.

Available devices include the Bonebridge™ (MED-EL, Innsbruck, Austria) [29], and the recently introduced Osia® 2 System (Cochlear Bone-Anchored Solutions AB, Mölnlycke, Sweden) [25]. The Bonebridge™ was first introduced in 2012 with the second version, the BCI602, released in 2019. The device is indicated for patients with CHL, MHL with BC PTA thresholds better than or equal to 45 dB HL, or SSD (Table 2; Figure 1). The implanted device consists of a magnet, receiving coil, demodulator which processes sounds, and an electromagnetic floating mass transducer (FMT) which generates mechanical vibrations [29]. The FMT is attached to the skull via cortical fixation screws that do not require osseointegration [43]. The BCI602 requires a bony recess drilled into the skull, though the BCI602 is smaller in size than the original implant making placement more straightforward. Optimal placement is in the pre-sigmoid mastoid bone. In patients that have had a prior mastoidectomy, alternative placement in a retrosigmoid position or above the temporal line may be required. The device has a flexible bridge between the receiver coil and the FMT to allow for greater flexibility in placement when needed. Lifts are available to limit the amount of required bone excavation and separate the device from underlying dura or sinuses [44,45]. Preoperative CT imaging is recommended [45]. The external processor is the SAMBA 2 processor which is held in place magnetically with six magnet strengths available [30]. With the external processor removed, this device is MRI compatible up to 1.5 Tesla (Table 3) [29].

The Osia® System was introduced in the United States in 2019 and indicated for patients with CHL, MHL with BC PTA thresholds of 55 dB HL or better, and SSD (Table 2; Figure 1) [25]. The system uses the same BI300 osseointegrated implant as other Cochlear™ devices with the OSI200 implant fixated to the osseointegrated BI300 screw [26]. Bone polishing may be required to ensure the transducer is in contact with the implant only and not surrounding bone, but drilling a bony well is not required [46]. This device uses a piezoelectric transducer which undergoes mechanical deformation when an electric voltage is applied [47]. This motion drives vibration through the BI300 implant to the skull, allowing for bone conduction hearing. The current device is not MRI compatible; the implanted magnet must be surgically removed before an MRI can be safely performed (Table 3) [27]. Available accessories and streaming capabilities are listed in Table 4.

3.2. Extrinsic Devices

Non-surgical bone conduction hearing devices are also available. These are attached to the patient via a headband, softband, adhesive, eyeglasses, or another mechanism. The external device is in contact with the skin, vibrates in response to sound, and transmits vibratory signals through the intact skin and soft tissue to the skull, leading to bone conduction hearing. These devices are subject to signal attenuation, especially at high frequencies, as the signal travels through soft tissue [7]. Depending on the attachment mechanism, the force required to hold the device in place and effectively transmit sound may limit wear time [48]. The same bone-anchored hearing processors used in the transcutaneous passive devices can be attached to a test band. Pre-implantation testing is recommended for patients considering bone-anchored hearing aid placement to help patients understand the benefits of such devices, sound quality, and the utility of choosing a bone conduction device.

Similar to passive transcutaneous devices, signal attenuation, especially at high frequencies, is expected [7]. Percutaneous or active transcutaneous devices would be expected to perform better, but the trial period allows patients to make a more informed decision about proceeding with surgery and the hearing quality they can anticipate post-operatively. Bone-anchored hearing aid placement is currently FDA-approved for children five years of age or older [49]. Children too young for implantation or adult patients for whom surgery is contraindicated may use a headband device as for amplification beyond the trial environment.

Previously introduced processors including Cochlear™ Baha® 5 series, Ponto 3 and 4 series, and Alpha MPO ePlus™ devices can all be worn externally on a soft band, headband, or other attachment mechanism. Two devices may be worn when bilateral amplification is indicated.

In addition to these devices, an adhesive option, the ADHEAR (MED-EL, Innsbruck, Austria) is also available [31]. This device is anchored with an adhesive applied to the skin over the mastoid bone which is designed to be worn for three to seven days. The audio processor connects to the adhesive and vibrates in response to sound, driving vibratory signal transmission through the skin and soft tissue to the underlying bone [31]. Since it is attached by an adhesive, pressure-induced discomfort is not a limitation to wear [48]. The ADHEAR is indicated for patients with unilateral or bilateral conductive hearing loss with a bone conduction HL better than or equal to 25 dB and for patients with single-sided deafness (Table 2; Figure 1) [31]. Available accessories and streaming capabilities are listed in Table 4.

The SoundBite (Sonitus Technologies, San Mateo, CA, USA) is a dental appliance designed to transmit vibratory signals to the skull via the teeth [50,51]. The device is not currently available, but a brief discussion is included here for reference. The device was designed for patients with single-sided deafness or conductive hearing loss with a bone conduction PTA better than or equal to 25 dB HL [20]. The SoundBite™ consists of an in-the-mouth (ITM) piezoelectric transducer placed on the buccal surface of the maxillary molars and a device worn on the poorer hearing ear which consists of a behind-the-ear (BTE) transducer and a microphone in the ear canal [51]. This has been found to be safe and uses forces far below those typically felt by the teeth during normal functions [50]. Production of the device stopped in 2015, but Sonitus Technologies was recently awarded a contract with the United States Department of Defense with the plan to rebrand the device as the Molar Mic™ for military personnel [52].

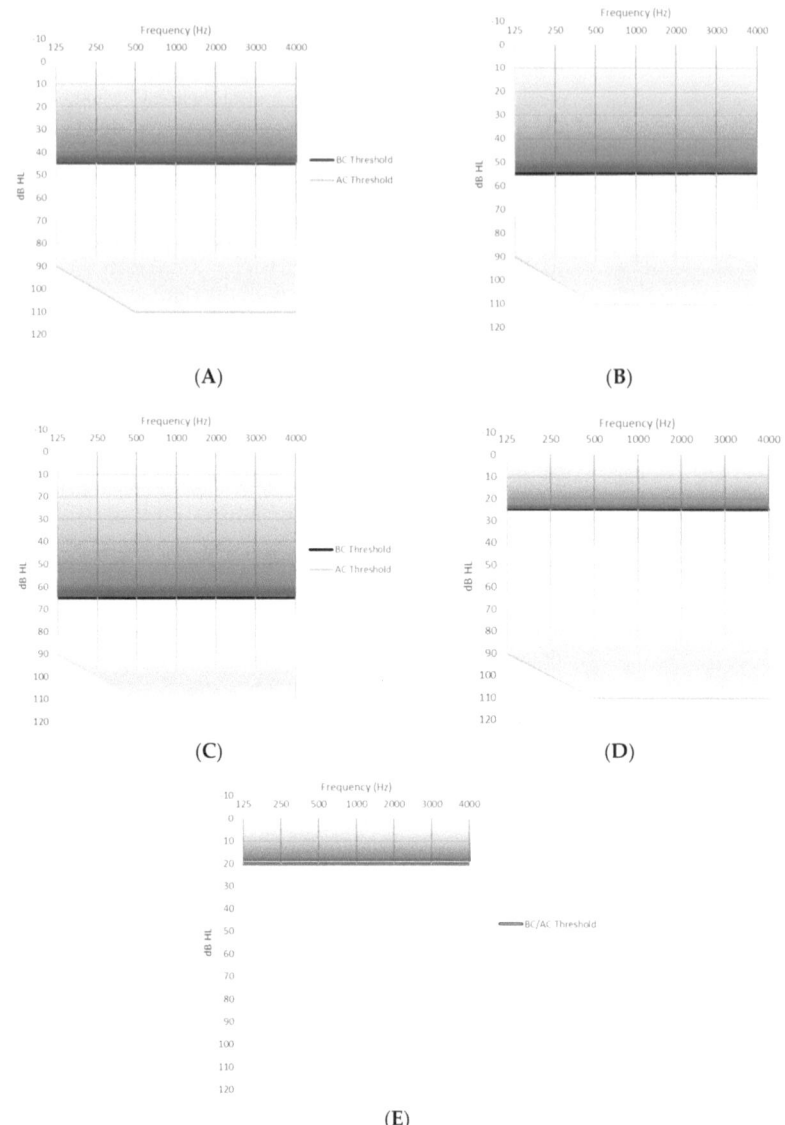

Figure 1. This figure depicts the fitting ranges for the described devices. The dark grey shaded area represents the range of recommended bone conduction thresholds in patients being considered for bone conduction hearing devices. The light grey shaded area demonstrates possible air conduction thresholds. (**A**) represents a 45 dB BC PTA, the recommended bone conduction hearing threshold for the Ponto 3 [15], Ponto 4 [15], Baha® 5 [17], Alpha 2 MPO ePlus™ [42], and SAMBA 2 [30] processors. (**B**) represents a 55 dB BC PTA, the recommended bone conduction hearing threshold for the Ponto 3 Power [15], Baha® 5 Power [17], Baha® 6 Max [16], and Osia® 2 [25] processors. (**C**) represents a 65 dB BC PTA, the recommended bone conduction hearing threshold for the Ponto 3 SueprPower [15] and the Baha® 5 SuperPower [17]. (**D**) represents a 25 dB BC PTA, the recommended bone conduction hearing threshold for the ADHEAR processor [31]. (**E**) represents a 20 dB BC PTA. For patients with SSD, the contralateral ear should have normal hearing—a BC and AC PTA of 20 dB or better. These figures were created from publicly available device information and reproduced with permission from Cochlear™, MED-EL, Medtronic, and Oticon representatives.

Table 3. Sound Processor Characteristics.

	Device	Processor	Size	Weight	Battery Type	Average Battery Life	IP Rating [53]
Percutaneous	Ponto [15,21]	Ponto 3	3.4 × 2.1 × 1.4 cm	14 g (without battery)	13	70–130 h	IP 57
		Ponto 3 Power	3.4 × 2.1 × 1.4 cm	17 g (without battery)	675	70–150 h	IP 57
		Ponto 3 Superpower	3.4 × 2.1 × 1.4 cm	17 g (without battery)	675 HP	35–80 h	IP 57
		Ponto 4	2.6 × 1.9 × 1.1 cm	13.2 g (without battery)	312	48–70 h	IP 57
	Baha® Connect [16,17,54,55]	Baha® 5	2.6 × 1.9 × 1.2 cm	9.8 g (without battery)	312	36–100 h	IP 63
		Baha® 5 Power	3.6 × 2.2 × 1.3 cm	17 g (without battery)	675	80–220 h	IP 63
		Baha® 5 SuperPower	3.9 × 4.8 × 0.9 cm	14.4 g (actuator); 9.8–12.7 g (processing unit + battery)	Rechargeable lithium	≤16 h (mini) ≤32 h (standard)	IP 63
		Baha® 6 Max	2.6 × 1.9 × 1.2 cm	11.5 g (without battery)	312	44–132 h	IP 68
Transcutaneous Passive	Alpha 2 MPO [23]	Alpha 2 MPO ePlus™	4.1 cm × 1.63 cm		13 or rechargeable	320 h or 32 h (rechargeable)	IP 22
	Baha® Attract [16,17,24]	Same as Baha® Connect				Same as above	
Transcutaneous Active	Osia® [22,25–27]	Osia® 2	3.6 × 3.2 × 1.04	7.8 g (with magnet; without battery)	675 HP		IP 52; IP 68 (with cover)
	Bonebridge™ [28–30]	SAMBA 2	3.0 × 3.5 × 1.0 cm	7.5 g (with magnet; without battery) *	675	133–210 h	IP 54; IP 68 (with cover)
Adhesive	ADHEAR [31]	ADHEAR	0.6 × 3.0 cm (adhesive) 1.5 × 3.5 cm (processor)	13.5 g (without battery)	13	Up to 300 h	

Device characteristics and compatibility for each processor are listed including external processor size, weight, battery type, battery life, and IP (ingress protection) rating. IP Rating = "ingress protection" rating, indicates the amount of resistance to solids and liquids. The first number indicates the amount of resistance to solids (with 0 being not protected, and 6 being dust-tight), and the second digit indicates the amount of resistance to liquids (with 0 being not protected, and 8 being protected from liquids up to 1m of submersion) [55]. Device information is included with permission from Cochlear™, MED-EL, Medtronic, and Oticon representatives. Note that battery life is variable depending on the programs and features utilized and streaming time. (HP = high power battery type). * D. Franz, email communication, April 2021.

Table 4. Sound Processor Connectivity and Accessories.

	Device	Processor	Wireless Accessories	Streaming Method	Direct iPhone Streaming	Direct Android Streaming
Percutaneous	Ponto [15,53,56]	Ponto 3 Ponto 3 Power Ponto 3 Superpower	Ponto 3 • Connect Line App • Oticon Medical Streamer on neck loop • Remote Mic • TV Adapter 2.0 • FM system compatible • Phone adapter 2.0 • BTD 500	NFMI on neck loop; 2.4 GHz to devices		
		Ponto 4	Ponto 4 • Oticon ON app • Remote Control 3.0 • Connect Clip (can be used as a remote mic) • TV Adapter 3.0 • Edumic • Phone adapter 2.0 • Bluetooth dongle • BTD 800	2.4 GHz	X	
	Baha® Connect [16,17,21,54,55,57]	Baha® 5, Baha® 5 Power, and Baha® 5 SuperPower	Baha 5 and 6 • Baha® Smart App • Remote Control 2 • Mini Microphone 2+ • Phone Clip • TV Streamer	2.4 GHz	X	
		Baha® 6 Max		2.4 GHz; Bluetooth LE	X	X
Transcutaneous Passive	Alpha 2 MPO [23]	Alpha 2 MPO ePlus™	None Note that DAI can be used for wired streaming and FM systems	DAI		
	Baha® Attract [7,16,17,24]	Baha® 5, Baha® 5 Power, and Baha® 5 SuperPower; Baha® 6 Max		Same as above		
Transcutaneous Active	Osia® [25–27,58]	Osia® 2	Osia® Smart App TrueWireless™ Phone Clip Mini mic 2 Remote control 2 TV streamer	2.4 GHz	X	
	BONEBRIDGE™ [9,28–30,59]	SAMBA 2	SAMBA2GO SAMBA 2 Remote App Note that DAI can be used for wired streaming and FM systems	NFMI on neck loop; Bluetooth or DAI to devices		
Adhesive	ADHEAR [31,60]	ADHEAR	None Note that DAI can be used for wired streaming and FM systems	DAI		

2.4 GHz = The 2.4 GHz Industrial Scientific Medical (ISM) band is similar to Bluetooth streaming and allows wireless signal to propagate through the air to connect/stream with the hearing processor. NFMI = near field magnetic induction; BT LE = Bluetooth low energy; Bluetooth technology that utilizes the traditional "frequency-hopping" 2.4 GHz band technology, but requires less energy consumption. Best for devices in short range of each other [61]. Device information is included with permission from Cochlear™, MED-EL, Medtronic, and Oticon representatives.

4. Conclusions

Since the introduction of bone conduction hearing technology, numerous devices have been developed to optimize signal transmission, limit skin and wound complications, and rehabilitate hearing for patients with conductive and mixed hearing loss and single-sided deafness. The recently introduced active transcutaneous devices, the Osia® and Bonebridge™, take advantage of new electronic signal transmission, optimize bone conduction efficiency, and reduce the incidence of skin complications. The current landscape of devices is described here and includes fitting criteria, patient selection, and benefits and drawbacks of each device. This condensed information is intended to be a resource for patients and providers alike to assist with proper device selection for each situation.

Author Contributions: Conceptualization, S.E.E., E.M.N., and E.Z.S.; methodology, S.E.E., E.M.N., and E.Z.S.; investigation, S.E.E., E.M.N., and E.Z.S.; resources, S.E.E. and E.M.N.; data curation, S.E.E., E.M.N., and E.Z.S.; writing—original draft preparation, S.E.E., E.M.N., and E.Z.S.; writing—review and editing, S.E.E., E.M.N., and E.Z.S.; visualization, S.E.E. and E.M.N.; supervision, E.Z.S. All authors have read and agreed to the published version of the manuscript.

Funding: This research received no external funding.

Institutional Review Board Statement: Not applicable.

Informed Consent Statement: Not applicable.

Acknowledgments: We would like to thank representatives from Cochlear™, MED-EL, Medtronic, and Oticon for providing device specifications and permission to reproduce this information in our review.

Conflicts of Interest: The authors declare no conflict of interest.

References

1. Mudry, A.; Tjellström, A. Historical background of bone conduction hearing devices and bone conduction hearing aids. *Adv. Otorhinolaryngol.* **2011**, *71*, 1–9.
2. Tjellström, A.; Lindström, J.; Hallén, O.; Albrektsson, T.; Brånemark, P.I. Osseointegrated titanium implants in the temporal bone. A clinical study on bone-anchored hearing aids. *Am. J. Otol.* **1981**, *2*, 304–310. [PubMed]
3. Brånemark, P.I.; Hansson, B.O.; Adell, R.; Breine, U.; Lindström, J.; Hallén, O.; Ohman, A. Osseointegrated implants in the treatment of the edentulous jaw. Experience from a 10-year period. *Scand. J. Plast Reconstr. Surg. Suppl.* **1977**, *16*, 1–132. [PubMed]
4. Dun, C.A.J.; Faber, H.T.; de Wolf, M.J.F.; Cremers, C.W.R.J.; Hol, M.K.S. An overview of different systems: The bone-anchored hearing aid. *Adv. Otorhinolaryngol.* **2011**, *71*, 22–31. [PubMed]
5. Stenfelt, S. Acoustic and physiologic aspects of bone conduction hearing. *Adv. Otorhinolaryngol.* **2011**, *71*, 10–21. [PubMed]
6. Stenfelt, S.; Goode, R.L. Bone-conducted sound: Physiological and clinical aspects. *Otol. Neurotol.* **2005**, *26*, 1245–1261. [CrossRef] [PubMed]
7. Verstraeten, N.; Zarowski, A.J.; Somers, T.; Riff, D.; Offeciers, E.F. Comparison of the audiologic results obtained with the bone-anchored hearing aid attached to the headband, the testband, and to the "snap" abutment. *Otol. Neurotol.* **2009**, *30*, 70–75. [CrossRef]
8. Calon, T.G.A.; Johansson, M.L.; de Brujin, A.J.; Berge, H.V.D.; Wagenaar, M.; Eichhorn, E.; Janssen, M.M.; Hof, J.R.; Brunings, J.-W.; Joore, M.A.; et al. Minimally invasive ponto surgery versus the linear incision technique with soft tissue preservation for bone conduction hearing implants: A multicenter randomized controlled trial. *Otol. Neurotol.* **2018**, *39*, 882–893. [CrossRef]
9. Høgsbro, M.; Agger, A.; Johansen, L.V. Successful loading of a bone-anchored hearing implant at two weeks after surgery: Randomized trial of two surgical methods and detailed stability measurements. *Otol. Neurotol.* **2015**, *36*, e51–e57. [CrossRef]
10. Høgsbro, M.; Agger, A.; Johansen, L.V. Successful Loading of a Bone-Anchored Hearing Implant at 1 Week After Surgery. *Otol. Neurotol.* **2017**, *38*, 207–211. [CrossRef]
11. McElveen, J.T., Jr.; Green, J.D., Jr.; Arriaga, M.A.; Slattery, W.H., 3rd. Next-Day Loading of a Bone-Anchored Hearing System: Preliminary Results. *Otolaryngol. Head Neck Surg.* **2020**, *163*, 582–587. [CrossRef] [PubMed]
12. Holgers, K.M.; Tjellström, A.; Bjursten, L.M.; Erlandsson, B.E. Soft tissue reactions around percutaneous implants: A clinical study of soft tissue conditions around skin-penetrating titanium implants for bone-anchored hearing aids. *Am. J. Otol.* **1998**, *9*, 56–59.
13. Mohamad, S.; Khan, I.; Hey, S.Y.; Hussain, S.S. A systematic review on skin complications of bone-anchored hearing aids in relation to surgical techniques. *Eur. Arch. Otorhinolaryngol.* **2016**, *273*, 559–565. [CrossRef] [PubMed]
14. Kiringoda, R.; Lustig, L.R. A meta-analysis of the complications associated with osseointegrated hearing aids. *Otol. Neurotol.* **2013**, *34*, 790–794. [CrossRef] [PubMed]
15. Candidacy Guide. Oticonmedical.com. 2017. Available online: https://www.oticonmedical.com/-/media/medical/main/files/for-professionals/bahs/audiological-materials/guide/eng/candidacy-guide---english---m52735.pdf?la=en-gb (accessed on 20 January 2021).
16. Cochlear. *Baha 6 Max Connect. Datasheet*; Cochlear Bone Anchored Solutions AB: Mölnlycke, Sweden, 2020.
17. Compare Baha® Sound Processors | Cochlear. Cochlear. 2018. Available online: https://www.cochlear.com/us/en/home/products-and-accessories/baha-system/baha-sound-processors/compare-baha-sound-processors (accessed on 22 January 2021).
18. Mylanus, E.A.; van der Pouw, K.C.; Snik, A.F.; Cremers, C.W. Intraindividual comparison of the bone-anchored hearing aid and air-conduction hearing aids. *Arch. Otolaryngol. Head Neck Surg.* **1998**, *124*, 271–276. [CrossRef] [PubMed]
19. Kruyt, I.J.; Nelissen, R.C.; Mylanus, E.A.M.; Hol, M.K.S. Three-year Outcomes of a Randomized Controlled Trial Comparing a 4.5-mm-Wide to a 3.75-mm-Wide Titanium Implant for Bone Conduction Hearing. *Otol. Neurotol.* **2018**, *39*, 609–615. [CrossRef]
20. Accessdata.fda.gov. 2011. Available online: https://www.accessdata.fda.gov/cdrh_docs/pdf11/K110831.pdf (accessed on 22 February 2021).

21. Oticon Ponto MRI Safety/Security Control Information. Oticonmedical.com. 2016. Available online: https://www.oticonmedical.com/-/media/medical/main/files/bahs/users-and-candidates/mri-security-card/eng/mri-security-card---english---m52283.pdf (accessed on 22 January 2021).
22. Cochlear™ Osia ® 2 Sound Processor User Manual. Cochlear.com. Available online: https://www.cochlear.com/e33e12e0-896e-4bac-baa3-f35683a95336/P1600518_D1600539-V2_Osia_2_SP_UM_EN_US.pdf?MOD=AJPERES (accessed on 10 March 2021).
23. Product Specification: Medtronic Alpha 2 MPO ePlus™. Asiapac.medtronic.com. 2017. Available online: https://asiapac.medtronic.com/content/dam/medtronic-com/us-en/patients/treatments-therapies/bone-conduction/documents/alpha-2-mpo-eplus-spec-sheet.pdf (accessed on 21 January 2021).
24. Cochlear™ Baha® Attract System: Radiographers Instructions for MRI. Cochlear.com. Published 2015. 2015. Available online: https://www.cochlear.com/f5917ef2-bb35-4307-b330-8c15ffdd993c/BUN264+ISS2+APR15+Baha+Attract+Radiographers+Instructions+for+MRI.pdf (accessed on 8 March 2021).
25. Cochlear™ Osia® System-Candidate Selection Guide. Cochlear.com. 2019. Available online: https://www.cochlear.com/2bae95f1-5a89-405c-8733-25d28b1e3c4e/OSI007-ISS1-DEC19-Osia-Candidate-Selection-Guide.pdf (accessed on 21 January 2021).
26. Technical Specifications: Cochlear™ Osia® 2 System. Cochlear.com. 2019. Available online: https://www.cochlear.com/b2f659ec-ca9a-4fad-b7a6-b929e6eaa078/OSI001-ISS1-NOV19-Osia-System-Tech-Spec.pdf (accessed on 8 March 2021).
27. Cochlear™ Osia® Magnetic Resonance Imaging (MRI) Guidelines. Cochlear.com. 2019. Available online: https://www.cochlear.com/ce7aa1b1-2862-4bcf-a9aa-491707b3556a/P1638364_D1638388-V3_Osia_MRI_Guidelines_EN-US%5B1%5D.pdf (accessed on 22 January 2021).
28. MRI Technologist's Guide: Medtronic Magnetic Implant Precautions. Medtronic.com. 2017. Available online: https://www.medtronic.com/content/dam/medtronic-com/us-en/patients/treatments-therapies/bone-conduction/documents/alpha-2-mpo-eplus-mri-tech-guide.pdf (accessed on 20 January 2021).
29. BCI 602: Active Bone Conduction Implant-BONEBRIDGE System. Sf.cdn.medel.com. 2019. Available online: https://sf.cdn.medel.com/docs/librariesprovider2/product/bci602/29214ce_r2_0-bci-602fs-web.pdf (accessed on 21 January 2021).
30. MED-EL. *BONEBRIDGE SAMBA 2 Audio Processor–Instructions for Use*; MED-EL: Innsbruck, Austria, 2020.
31. ADHEAR System-Including the ADHEAR Audio Processor and the ADHEAR Adhesive Adapter. S3.medel.com. Available online: https://s3.medel.com/pdf/28867_30_ADHEAR_Factsheet-EN.pdf (accessed on 23 January 2021).
32. Surgery Guide: A Bone Conduction Hearing Solution-Cochlear™ Baha® DermaLock™ Surgical Procedure. Cochlear.com. 2015. Available online: https://www.cochlear.com/66b43e66-3e0b-453b-9751-bc904f3961fd/BUN128+ISS4+NOV30+-+Baha+Connect+Surgery+Guide+FINAL.pdf (accessed on 8 March 2021).
33. Chen, S.; Mancuso, D.; Lalwani, A. Skin Necrosis After Implantation with the BAHA Attract: A Case Report and Review of the Literature. *Otol Neurotol.* **2017**, *38*, 364–367. [CrossRef]
34. Cooper, T.; McDonald, B.; Ho, A. Passive Transcutaneous Bone Conduction Hearing Implants: A Systematic Review. *Otol. Neurotol.* **2017**, *38*, 1225–1232. [CrossRef]
35. Surgery Guide: Cochlear™ Baha® Attract System Surgical Procedure. Cochlear.com. 2017. Available online: https://www.cochlear.com/5e7d4527-a3c0-4b19-8814-e7494fdaba07/BUN226-ISS4-APR17-Baha-Attract-Surgery-Guide.pdf (accessed on 8 March 2021).
36. den Betsen, C.A.; Monksfuekd, P.; Bosman, A.; Skarzynski, P.H.; Green, K.; Runge, C.; Wigren, S.; Blechert, J.I.; Flynn, M.C.; Mylanus, E.A.M.; et al. Audiological and clinical outcomes of a transcutaneous bone conduction hearing implant: Six-month results from a multicentre study. *Clin. Otolaryngol.* **2019**, *44*, 144–157.
37. Hol, M.K.; Nelissen, R.C.; Agterberg, M.J.; Cremers, C.W.; Snik, A.F. Comparison between a new implantable transcutaneous bone conductor and percutaneous bone-conduction hearing implant. *Otol. Neurotol.* **2013**, *34*, 1071–1075. [CrossRef]
38. Kurz, A.; Flynn, M.; Caversaccio, M.; Kompis, M. Speech understanding with a new implant technology: A comparative study with a new nonskin penetrating Baha system. *Biomed. Res. Int.* **2014**, *2014*, 416205. [CrossRef] [PubMed]
39. Cochlear™ Baha® Attract System: Sound Processor Magnet Selection Guide. Cochlear.com. 2016. Available online: https://www.cochlear.com/d41ece87-f6a5-44e3-8f94-53dd6a77edcd/BUN225-ISS3-SEP16-Baha-Attract-SP-Magnet-Selection-Guide.pdf (accessed on 22 January 2021).
40. Cedars, E.; Chan, D.; Lao, A.; Hardies, L.; Meyer, A.; Rosbe, K. Conversion of traditional osseointegrated bone-anchored hearing aids to the Baha® attract in four pediatric patients. *Int. J. Pediatr. Otorhinolaryngol.* **2016**, *91*, 37–42. [CrossRef] [PubMed]
41. Bere, Z.; Vass, G.; Perenyi, A.; Tobias, Z.; Rovo, L. Surgical Solution for the Transformation of the Percutaneous Bone Anchored Hearing Aid to a Transcutaneous System in Complicated Cases. *J. Int. Adv. Otol.* **2020**, *16*, 477–481. [CrossRef] [PubMed]
42. Alpha 2 MPO ePLUS™ Candidacy Guide. Medtronic.com. 2017. Available online: https://www.medtronic.com/content/dam/medtronic-com/us-en/patients/treatments-therapies/bone-conduction/documents/alpha-2-mpo-eplus-candidacy-guide.pdf (accessed on 21 January 2021).
43. Sprinzl, G.M.; Wolf-Magele, A. The Bonebridge bone conduction hearing implant: Indication criteria, surgery, and a systemic review of the literature. *Clin. Otolaryngology.* **2016**, *42*, 131–143. [CrossRef]
44. Oh, S.J.; Goh, E.K.; Choi, S.W.; Lee, S.; Lee, H.-M.; Lee, I.-W.; Kong, S.-K. Audiologic, surgical and subjective outcomes of active transcutaneous bone conduction implant system (Bonebridge). *Int. J. Audiol.* **2019**, *58*, 956–963. [CrossRef]
45. Carnevale, C.; Thomás-Barberán, M.; Til-Pérez, G.; Sarría-Echegaray, P. The Bonebridge active bone conduction system: A fast and safe technique for a middle fossa approach. *J. Laryngol. Otol.* **2019**, *133*, 344–347. [CrossRef]

46. Mylanus, E.A.M.; Hua, H.; Wigren, S.; Arndt, S.; Skarzynski, P.H.; Telian, S.A.; Briggs, R.J.S. Multicenter Clinical Investigation of a New Active Osseointegrated Steady-State Implant System. *Otol. Neurotol.* **2020**, *41*, 1249–1257. [CrossRef]
47. Calero, D.; Paul, S.; Gesing, A.; Alves, F.; Cordioli, J.A. A technical review and evaluation of implantable sensors for hearing devices. *BioMed Eng. OnLine.* **2018**, *17*, 1–23. [CrossRef]
48. Skarzynski, P.H.; Ratuszniak, A.; Osinska, K.; Koziel, M.; Krol, B.; Cywka, K.B.; Skarzynski, H. A Comparative Study of a Novel Adhesive Bone Conduction Device and Conventional Treatment Options for Conductive Hearing Loss. *Otol. Neurotol.* **2019**, *40*, 858–864. [CrossRef]
49. Accessdata.fda.gov. 2016. Available online: https://www.accessdata.fda.gov/cdrh_docs/pdf16/K161123.pdf (accessed on 24 January 2021).
50. Popelka, G.R.; Derebery, J.; Blevins, N.H.; Murray, M.; Moore, B.C.; Sweetow, R.W.; Wu, B.; Katsis, M. Preliminary evaluation of a novel bone-conduction device for single-sided deafness. *Otol. Neurotol.* **2010**, *31*, 492–497. [CrossRef]
51. Gurgel, R.K.; Shelton, C. The SoundBite hearing system: Patient-assessed safety and benefit study. *Laryngoscope* **2013**, *123*, 2807–2812. [CrossRef] [PubMed]
52. Sonitus Technologies Wins Multi-Million Dollar DOD Award for 'Molar Mic'. 11 September 2018. Available online: http://www.sonitustechnologies.com/sonitus-technologies-wins-multi-million-dollar-dod-award-for-molar-mic/ (accessed on 22 February 2021).
53. IEC 60529. *Degrees of Protection Provided by Enclosures (IP Codes)*; International Electrotechnical Commision: Geneva, Switzerland, 2011.
54. Cochlear™ Baha® Connect System: Radiographers Instructions for MRI. Cochlear.com. 2015. Available online: https://www.cochlear.com/107fc39f-bf96-47b6-9527-7d603b654344/BUN380+ISS1+AUG15+Radiographers+Instructions.pdf (accessed on 8 March 2021).
55. Datasheet: Cochlear™ Baha® 6 Max Sound Processor. Cochlear.com. BUN871 ISS1 FEB21. Available online: https://www.cochlear.com/d6cd6d3d-8c98-4fae-b0aa-8a6bcaba405e/BUN871+Cochlear+Baha+6+Max+DataSheet+ISS1.pdf?MOD=AJPERES&CVID=nxbWkhz (accessed on 10 March 2021).
56. Featured Accessories. Oticon Medical. 2021. Available online: https://www.oticonmedical.com/us/bone-conduction/solutions/accessories (accessed on 10 March 2021).
57. Baha Accessories. Cochlear.com. 2020. Available online: https://store.mycochlear.com/store/index.php/aub2c/baha-implants.html (accessed on 10 March 2021).
58. Osia® Smartphone Compatibility. Cochlear.Com. 2019. Available online: https://www.cochlear.com/us/en/home/products-and-accessories/cochlear-osia-system/osia-2/osia-smartphone-compatibility (accessed on 10 March 2021).
59. MED-EL. *SAMBA 2 GO–Instructions for Use*; MED-EL: Innsbruck, Austria, 2020.
60. MED-EL. *ADHEAR: A Revolution in Bone Conduction Technology. Connectivity Information Provided by MED-EL*; MED-EL: Innsbruck, Austria, 2020.
61. Siekkinen, M.; Hiienkari, M.; Nurminen, J.K.; Nieminen, J. How low energy is bluetooth low energy? Comparative measurements with ZigBee/802.15.4. In Proceedings of the 2012 IEEE Wireless Communications and Networking Conference Workshops (WCNCW), Paris, France, 14 April 2012; pp. 232–237. [CrossRef]

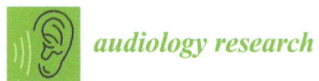

Article

Audiological Performance of ADHEAR Systems in Simulated Conductive Hearing Loss: A Case Series with a Review of the Existing Literature

Enrico Muzzi [1,†], Valeria Gambacorta [2,*,†], Ruggero Lapenna [2,†], Giulia Pizzamiglio [1], Sara Ghiselli [1], Igor Caregnato [3], Raffaella Marchi [1], Giampietro Ricci [2] and Eva Orzan [1]

[1] Audiology and Otorhinolaryngology Unit, Institute for Maternal and Child Health-Istituto di Ricerca a Carattere Clinico e Scientifico "Burlo Garofolo", 34137 Trieste, Italy; enrico.muzzi@burlo.trieste.it (E.M.); giuliapizzamiglio93@gmail.com (G.P.); S.Ghiselli@ausl.pc.it (S.G.); raffaella.marchi@burlo.trieste.it (R.M.); eva.orzan@burlo.trieste.it (E.O.)
[2] Department of Surgical and Biomedical Sciences, Section of Otorhinolaryngology, University of Perugia, 06129 Perugia, Italy; ruggerolapenna@gmail.com (R.L.); giampietro.ricci@unipg.it (G.R.)
[3] Acustica Caregnato, 36063 Marostica, Italy; igor.caregnato@gmail.com
* Correspondence: gambacortavaleria@gmail.com
† Enrico Muzzi, Valeria Gambacorta, Ruggero Lapenna equally contributed.

Abstract: A new non-invasive adhesive bone conduction hearing device (ABCD) has been proposed as an alternative solution for reversible bilateral conductive hearing loss in recurrent or long-lasting forms of otitis media with effusion (OME) in children that cannot undergo surgical treatment. Our aim was to assess the effectiveness of ABCD in children with OME. Twelve normal-hearing Italian-speaking volunteers, in whom a conductive hearing loss was simulated, participated in the study. The free-field average hearing threshold was determined and, to evaluate binaural hearing skills, loudness summation and the squelch effect were assessed. Five conditions were tested: (1) unaided without earplugs, (2) unaided with bilateral earplugs, (3) aided right ear with bilateral earplugs, (4) aided left ear with bilateral earplugs, and (5) bilateral aid with bilateral earplugs. Post-hoc analysis showed a significant statistical difference between plugged, unplugged, and each aided condition. The main results were a better loudness summation and a substantial improvement of the squelch effect in the bilaterally aided. Our results suggest that ABCD is a valid treatment for patients with conductive hearing loss that cannot undergo bone conduction implant surgery. It is also important to consider bilateral aids in order to deal with situations in which binaural hearing is fundamental.

Keywords: conductive hearing loss; bone conduction hearing device; otitis media with effusion; binaural hearing

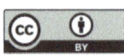

1. Introduction

Purely conductive hearing loss is determined by a decrease of the middle ear capacity to transmit sound to the normal inner ear. It can be congenital (e.g., external and/or middle ear malformations), or acquired either during childhood or during the adult life. These last forms are mainly due to inflammatory processes of the middle ear, and they can be permanent (e.g., following ossicular chain erosion due to cholesteatoma) or reversible/fluctuant.

The most representative situation giving a (potentially) reversible bilateral conductive hearing loss is the so-called "otitis media with effusion" (OME). It affects about 90% of children before school age [1], with the highest prevalence rates between 6 months and 4 years of age. Although most episodes of OME resolve spontaneously within 3 months, 30–40% of children experience recurrent events, and in 5 to 10% of cases, last more than one year [2].

When middle ear effusion persists for a long period of time, it can cause a significant decrease in hearing sensitivity, which could result in impaired school performance, failure to respond appropriately to normal conversational speech or environmental sounds, behavioral changes, and possibly a negative impact on the child's normal speech development [3,4].

Middle ear effusion generally results in a mild conductive hearing loss [5] of approximately 18–35 dB HL [6]. About 50% of patients with a confirmed OME diagnosis present a hearing loss of 20 dB, 20% a hearing loss greater than 35 dB, and 5–10% hearing loss of up to 50 dB [5]. In case of particularly recurrent or long-lasting forms of OME, the insertion of tympanic ventilation tubes (VTs) is considered to be the gold standard treatment VT to significantly improve hearing and reduce the number of OME while in place [2]. However, there are children with specific situations, such as syndromes (e.g., Down S.) or craniofacial disorders, that could have a high anesthesia risk or also a greater recurrence possibility after VT extrusion that does not suggest VT as the best treatment choice. In these patients, hearing aids, and specifically bone conduction devices, represent the alternative solution for the hearing problem. This option gives an excellent audiological benefit but presents disadvantages.

Recently, a new non-invasive adhesive bone conduction hearing device (ABCD) was proposed to overcome some of the disadvantages of previous disposable bone conduction hearing aids, such as bulkiness and pressure annoyance, with general poor acceptance by the child and the parents [7]. ABCD could potentially be suitable for temporary conductive hearing loss for cases in which surgical treatment cannot be proposed, failed, or should be postponed. Previous studies about ABCD are not very numerous; they deal both with real and simulated conductive hearing loss, both bilateral and unilateral forms, both in the adult and in the children population.

In this paper, we report our experience with the ABCD in a series of subjects with simulated conductive hearing loss with particular reference to binaural listening abilities with unilateral and bilateral aid use.

2. Materials and Methods
2.1. Study Subjects and Test Device

Twelve normal-hearing Italian-speaking volunteers, four males and eight females, with a mean age of 31.2 years (range 23–45) participated in the study. In order to simulate a mild-to-moderate bilateral conductive hearing loss, external ear canals were occluded with customized silicone earplugs. Two subjects left the study before completing all the measurements. The ABCD system (ADHEAR, MedEl, Innsbruck, Austria) is a commercially available bone conduction hearing device retained by an advanced adhesive adapter on the hairless skin over the mastoid. The optimal position of the device in the retro auricular area was identified, making sure to avoid contact with the pinna; cleansed and gently rubbed with 70° alcohol; and the adhesive adapter was placed by exerting a slight pressure. The position on the skull should fit the curvature of the adapter well, maximizing the adhesive surface, without any hair underneath

It should be noted that the ABCD is reversible in order to be applied either on the left or on the right but not symmetrical, i.e., the microphone is located in the upper part of the device when applied on the left and in the lower part of the device when placed on the right (Figure 1).

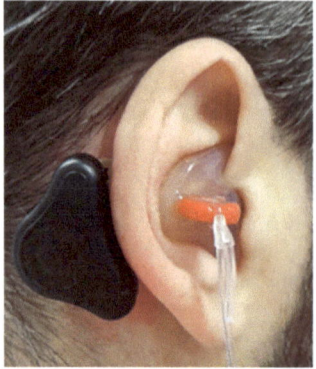
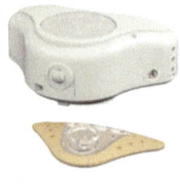

Figure 1. Right ear. ABCD device in place in a typical subject, where the ear canal is occluded by a custom silicone plug. On the right, a commercial figure of the ABCD showing the external laterale surface is visible, and the microphone ports are visible on the right (in the lower part of the device when worn on the right side).

2.2. Hearing Tests

The free-field average hearing threshold at 0.5, 1, 2, and 4 kHz was determined using narrowband noise (NBN) stimuli.

The speech signal consisted of random phonetically balanced lists of 20 spondaic words in the Italian language [8] delivered at 50 dB HL, while pink noise was used as a masker. With the aim of evaluating binaural hearing skills, loudness summation and the squelch effect were tested. To evaluate loudness summation, speech and noise were presented from the same loudspeaker located frontally (Figure 2A). For measuring the squelch effect, both conditions were tested with noise from the right side (+90°, Figure 2B) and from the left side (−90°, Figure 2C), while speech was presented from the front. An adaptive procedure with 2 dB increments/decrements of noise starting from a signal-to-noise ratio (SNR) of 10 dB was employed. The speech reception threshold corresponding to 50% of word recognition (SRT_{50}) was taken as the reference target. Overall "best scenario" and "worst scenario" SRT_{50} scores were those obtained in case of unilateral aid use in the conditions of noise lateralized to the unaided side or to the aided side, respectively. The lower the value of SRT_{50}, the better the hearing performance in noise.

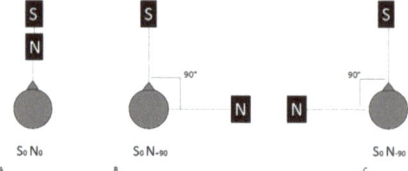

Figure 2. Speech-in-noise test setup. S, signal (speech) source location, N, noise source location. (**A**) Loudness summation test; (**B**) Right squelch effect test; (**C**) Left squelch effect test.

Tests were carried out in a soundproof audiometric booth, with loudspeakers positioned at a distance of 1 m from the subject, at the level of the ears. The subjects were advised to avoid head movements during the test. Five conditions were tested: (1) unaided without earplugs, (2) unaided with bilateral earplugs, (3) aided right ear with bilateral earplugs, (4) aided left ear with bilateral earplugs, and (5) bilateral aid with bilateral earplugs.

2.3. Statistical Analysis

Results are presented as aided and unaided frequency-specific thresholds expressed as mean values ± SD or median and quartiles (q1; q3) as indicated. The patients' comparisons were evaluated using two-way ANOVA with post hoc analysis with Tukey test for free field NBN hearing thresholds. Wilcoxon rank sum test (with Bonferroni correction for multiple comparison to avoid type I error) was used to compare SNR50 values with different aided conditions in each tested hearing in noise situation. p values < 0.05 were considered significant. Data were analyzed using Excel (version 16.23) and R Commander (version 3.6.0 GUI 1.70) for IOS 10.14.4.

3. Results

3.1. Free Field Average Hearing Threshold

Figure 3 shows the mean free field threshold in each test condition.

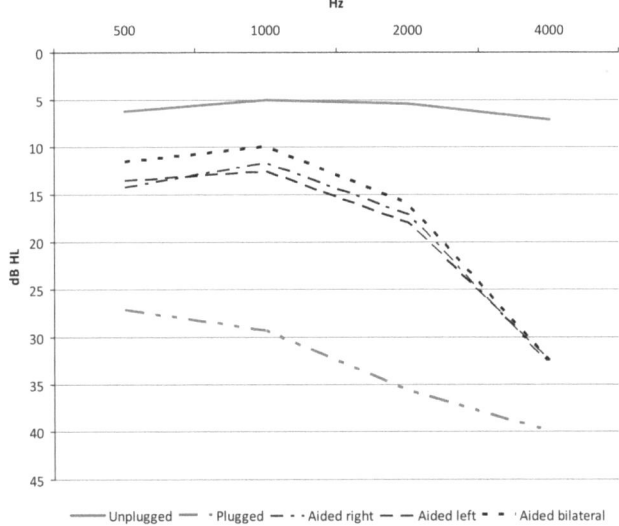

Figure 3. Average free-field threshold in each test condition.

Mean value ± SD values are shown in Table 1.

Table 1. Free Field NBN audiometry results for tested frequencies in each condition.

	500 Hz	1000 Hz	2000 Hz	4000 Hz
Unplugged	6.25 ± 2.26	5 ± 3	5.42 ± 3.96	7.08 ± 3.34
Plugged	28.3 ± 6.85	27.14 ± 7.48	36.25 ± 6.9	42.5 ± 6.9
Aided right	14.17 ± 2.8	11.67 ± 3.25	17.08 ± 3.96	32.92 ± 4.98
Aided left	13.5 ± 2.4	12.5 ± 3.5	18 ± 3.5	32.5 ± 5.9
Aided bil	11.5 ± 3.37	10 ± 2.35	16 ± 5.6	32.5 ± 4.24

Given the values of the average NBN audiometry (500, 1000, 2000, 4000 Hz) with plugged ear, post hoc analysis of the power of the sample with respect to the OME population showed a value of 89.1%.

There was a statistically significant main effect of condition and frequency for the studied audiometry thresholds (two-way ANOVA; $p < 0.0001$). Post-hoc analysis showed a statistically significant difference between the unplugged and plugged conditions, between the plugged and each aided condition, and also between the unplugged and each aided condition (Tukey's test; $p < 0.01$). No statistically significant differences were found between the three different aided conditions (Tukey's test; $p > 0.05$). Although there was no difference between the thresholds at each of the frequencies in the unplugged condition (Tukey's test; $p > 0.05$), there were a statistically significantly higher threshold for 2–4 kHz than 0.5–1 kHz in each study condition (Tukey's test; $p < 0.01$). However, there was a statistically significant gain for each frequency in the aided conditions (Tukey's test; $p < 0.01$)

3.2. Binaural Hearing in Noise (Loudness Summation and Squelch Effect)

The median SRT_{50} values (interquartile range) for the loudness summation (S_0N_0) and squelch effect (S_0N_{+90} and S_0N_{-90}) testing are reported in Table 2.

Table 2. Median SNR_{50} values (interquartile range) at loudness summation (S_0N_0) and squelch effect (S_0N_{+90} and S_0N_{-90}) testing.

	Loudness Summation S_0N_0	Squelch Effect (S_0N_{+90})	Squelch Effect (S_0N_{-90})
Unplugged	2 dB (0; 2.3)	−5 dB (−7; −2)	−2 dB (−3.5; −1)
Plugged	4.5 dB (3.8; 7)	3 dB (2; 5)	3 dB (0.75; 5)
Aided right	3 dB (3; 6.3)	4 dB (3; 6)	0 dB (−1; 1.5)
Aided left	5.5 dB (4; 7.8)	0 dB (0; 2),	5 dB (2.25; 5.75)
Aided bil	3 dB (2.3; 4.8)	0 dB (−4; 3)	1 dB (−1.5; 3.5)

3.2.1. Loudness Summation S_0N_0

There is a statistically significant difference for the SRT_{50} values between the unplugged and plugged conditions ($p < 0.0125$; Wilcoxon rank sum test with Bonferroni correction). The greatest improvement is reached with the bilaterally aided condition, even if a clear statistical significance is not reached ($p = 0.051$; Figure 4). However, SRT_{50} with the bilateral aid does not statistically differ from the unplugged condition, while SRT_{50} is statistically significantly higher for both unilateral aided conditions with respect to the unplugged one ($p < 0.0125$).

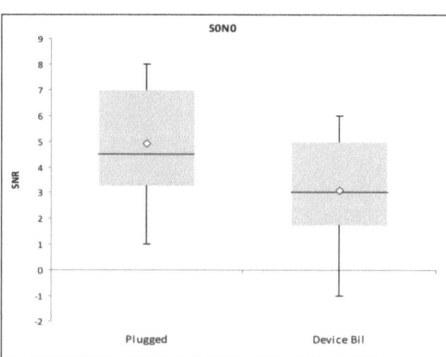

Figure 4. Loudness summation SRT_{50} for the unaided and bilaterally aided plugged condition.

3.2.2. Squelch Effect (S_0N_{+90})

There is a statistically significant difference for the SRT_{50} values between the unplugged and plugged conditions ($p < 0.0125$; Wilcoxon rank sum test with Bonferroni correction). A statistically significant improvement compared to the plugged condition is reached only in the bilaterally aided condition ($p < 0.0125$; Wilcoxon rank sum test with Bonferroni correction). SRT_{50} with the bilateral aid and with the aid on the left (best scenario) is not statistically different from the unplugged condition ($p > 0.0125$). SRT_{50} is statistically significantly higher for the right aided condition (worst scenario; $p < 0.0125$)

compared both to the unplugged condition and to the bilaterally aided one ($p < 0.0125$; Wilcoxon rank sum test with Bonferroni correction).

3.2.3. Squelch Effect (S_0N_{-90})

There is a statistically significant difference for the SRT_{50} values between the unplugged and plugged conditions ($p < 0.0125$; Wilcoxon rank sum test with Bonferroni correction). The greatest improvement is reached with the bilaterally aided condition, even if a clear statistical significance is not reached ($p = 0.09$). SRT_{50} with the bilateral aid and with the aid on the right (best scenario) is not statistically different from the unplugged condition ($p > 0.0125$). SNR_{50} is statistically significantly higher for the left aided condition (worst scenario; $p < 0.0125$) compared both to the unplugged condition and to the bilaterally aided one ($p < 0.0125$; Wilcoxon rank sum test with Bonferroni correction).

Figure 5 graphically shows the overall SRT_{50} scores in the aided conditions in the different situations of noise localization. It can be seen that there is a worsening of SRT50 in the worst noise source scenario compared to the plugged condition.

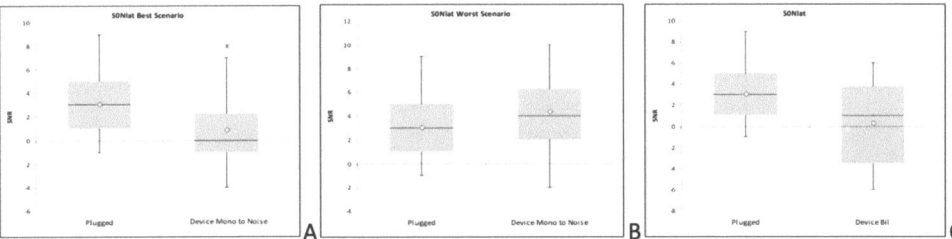

Figure 5. Aided squelch SRT50. (**A**) Overall scores with noise lateralized to the unaided ear, or "best scenario"; (**B**) Overall scores with noise lateralized to the aided ear, or "worst scenario"; (**C**) Overall bilaterally aided condition.

4. Discussion

The benefit derived from ABCD when compared to the simulated unaided conductive hearing loss measurements is clear.

In the present paper, we simulated bilateral conductive hearing loss in normal hearing subjects to assess the effectiveness of ABCD, for example, in children with OME, which potentially leads to a poorer quality of life in the patient and could negatively influence daily life, especially when binaural hearing is necessary (e.g., school).

Air conduction hearing devices have been traditionally successfully adopted in cases of CHL due to chronic or particularly recurrent forms of OME. However, bone conduction hearing aids overcome some disadvantages of external ear canal occlusion, allowing the necessity of regulation of the gain in relation to the possible fluctuation of the air-bone gap to be avoided. In the presence of normal bone conduction, BC hearing aids do not necessitate any regulation due to the different aid conduction threshold at any time.

The study was conducted in young adults because of the number of tests conducted that would not be tolerated by children. The conclusions are supposed to be relevant for children with bilateral conductive hearing loss as well because even if young children need a more favorable signal-to-noise ratio than adults [9], the OME-related hearing loss simulation method in children leads to a comparable speech perception impairment [10].

Other studies have demonstrated that speech perception performance in children with simulated hearing impairment is similar to that of children with OME [6]. Therefore, the simulated conductive hearing loss can be used to compare the hearing abilities and potential speech perception impairment of children with OME. We successfully simulated a mild to moderate hearing loss (average 33.75 dB HL), in a range similar to what is expected in case of OME (18–35 dB HL) using an earplug. Then, we tested hearing abilities in noise and in quiet environments.

With reference to the free field NBN hearing thresholds, a significant difference between the unplugged and plugged conditions and between plugged and each of the aided conditions was observed. Instead, there was no difference in the hearing threshold between the aided conditions. There was also a difference in the gain obtained with the use of ABCD for the individual frequencies. A better gain was observed in the low and mid frequencies compared to 4 kHz. Previous studies about ABCD application in CHL [11,12] obtained similar results. This means that normal hearing is still better than the aided one and that limitations of transcutaneous bone conduction are still present.

Most previous studies about ABCD application were heterogeneous regarding the included subjects (age and hearing loss etiology), ABCD side application procedure, and hearing abilities tested.

The main novelty of this study was testing the binaural hearing abilities in different experimental situations, including the bilaterally aided condition and different combinations of noise sources when testing the hearing in noise ability. The main results were a better loudness summation and a substantial improvement of the squelch effect in the bilaterally aided condition compared to the other conditions tested.

Binaural hearing is based on spatial auditory cues, such as interaural time difference and interaural level difference between the two ears, that can help a human localize the sound source. In case of binaural impairment, skills, such as recognizing speech in noise or localizing the direction of sound, become more difficult. For this reason, Snapp et al. [13] stated that bilateral hearing stimulation is considered the gold standard to achieve excellent auditory performance.

Bilateral bone conduction hearing aid application (e.g., ABCD) in case of bilateral conductive hearing loss allows binaural hearing to be restored and overcomes such environmental noise situations in which a unilateral hearing aid would be paradoxically disadvantageous (e.g., the noise source on the side of the hearing aid). In this sense, our study confirms Neumann et al.'s findings [14].

Other studies about ABCD [12,15–17] also compared them to conventional bone conduction hearing aids (BCHAs) in subjects with true or simulated conductive hearing loss. They found that audiologic assessment of aided sound field thresholds, SRTs in quiet and in noise, and WRSs showed no statistically significant differences when comparing the two devices. In particular, the ABCD also showed better results than the BCHA on a soft-band and therefore seems to be a promising solution for children with CHL aged below 10 years [14]. Comparing ABCD and BCHA, a statistically significant difference concerning daily usage was also found: the median reported wearing time of the adhesive device was 8.1 h compared to 4.3 h of conventional BCHA usage [15].

ABCD is a safe and effective device to treat conductive hearing loss and may considerably improve the quality of life for patients affected by OME. This device is well tolerated, its pressure-free nature could be an advantage over the other BCHA, causing no pain or skin irritation for the majority of patients.

However, the literature shows some limits of this device. Dahm et al. estimated an average battery durability of 5.9 days [11], but as stated by Neumann et al., excessive handling of the adapter, mastoid shape, skin type, and sweating could cause variation [14]. As stated by Mertens et al., for optimal retention of the adhesive adapter, special attention should be paid to the skin preparation (clean and dry) and correct placement [18].

For scientific and consultation purposes, a comprehensive review of the existing literature about ABCD is reported in Table 3.

Table 3. Comprehensive review of the existing literature about ABCD.

Authors	Subjects	Aided Condition Tested	Tests	Results
Brill et al. 2019 [19]	N = 12 Age = Adult Simulated with bilateral conductive hearing loss with a foam earplug	Unilateral ABCD.	- Free field tone audiometry - Number perception - Monosyllable perception	- Improvement in free-field hearing thresholds and significant tone audiometry gain.
Weiss et al. 2019 [20]	N = 11 Age = 18 years of age or older. Transient conductive hearing loss due to auditory canal tamponade after middle ear surgery.	Unilateral ABCD at the tamponade side, with contralateral ear plugged and covered.	- Free field tone audiometry. - Speech reception thresholds (SRT) in quiet and SRT in noise S_0N_0. - Speech, Spatial, and Qualities of Hearing 12 questionnaire.	- Speech perception for monosyllables in quiet improved. - Functional hearing gain improved. - Speech perception in noise improved. - The results of the questionnaire showed a high level of patient satisfaction and subjective hearing improvement.
Almuhawas et al. 2020 [21]	N = 12 Age = between 5 and 53 years. Conductive hearing loss (different etiologies).	Unilateral ABCD with the contralateral ear occluded with specific earplugs.	- Free field tone audiometry. - Speech reception threshold in quiet and noise. - Speech, Spatial, and Qualities of Hearing 12 questionnaire (SSQ12).	- Overall improvement in the aided thresholds when compared to the unaided hearing thresholds in the sound field. - Significant difference in speech perception in free field - Significantly higher word recognition scores in the aided condition - The results of the patient surveys using SSQ12 questionnaires demonstrated improved auditory performance hearing sensation and a high satisfaction rate for the system
Dahm et al. 2018 [11]	N = 12 Age = between 14 to 74 years. Bilateral or unilateral conductive hearing loss (different etiologies).	Unilateral ABCD, with the contralateral ear covered with a circumaural earmuff or with the application of a masking signal.	- Free field tone audiometry - Speech reception threshold (SRT) in quiet and in noise - Speech, Spatial, and Qualities of Hearing 12 questionnaire.	- Hearing gain at free field audiometry and SRT. - The sound field comparison to a conventional softband BCHA showed comparable levels of benefit.
Dahm et al. 2019 [15]	N = 13 Age = between 12 to 63 years Unilateral or bilateral conductive hearing loss	Unilateral ABCD, with the application in the contralateral ear of a masking signal Unilateral BCHA, with the application in the contralateral ear of a masking signal.	- Free field tone audiometry. - Speech reception threshold in quiet and in noise. - Speech, Spatial, and Qualities of Hearing 12 questionnaire. - Assessment of Quality of Life-8 Dimensions questionnaire.	- Statistically significant difference concerning the daily usage between an ABCD and a BCHA. - No statistically significant audiological difference between the two devices.
Favoreel et al. 2020 [16]	N = 10 Age = between 4 to 17 years. Unilateral or bilateral conductive hearing loss.	Unilateral ABCD with contralateral ear closed with an earplug and headphones. Unilateral BCHA with contralateral ear closed with an earplug and headphones.	- Free field tone audiometry. - Speech audiometry in quiet. - Speech, Spatial, and Qualities of Hearing 12 questionnaire.	- Hearing improvements with the ABCD and the BCHA on a softband. - No significant difference between the ABCD and the BCHA.

Table 3. Cont.

Authors	Subjects	Aided Condition Tested	Tests	Results
Kuthubutheen et al. 2020 [12]	N = 12 Age = between 11 to 70 years. Unilateral conductive hearing loss.	Unilateral ABCD. Unilateral BCHA.	- Free field tone audiometry. - Speech audiometry in quiet and in noise (S_0N_0). - Speech, Spatial, and Qualities of Hearing 12 questionnaire.	- Significant improvements in pure-tone thresholds as well as speech understanding both in quiet and in noise with both devices.
Neumann et al. 2019 [14]	N = 10 Age = between 3 months to 10 years. Unilateral or bilateral conductive hearing loss.	Unilateral ABCD, with the application in the contralateral ear of a masking signal. Unilateral BCHA with the application in the contralateral ear of a masking signal.	- Free field tone audiometry. - Speech audiometry in quiet and in noise. - LittlEARS Auditory Questionnaire. - Speech, Spatial and Qualities of Hearing Scale Questionnaire for parents.	- Functional gain with the ABCD exceeded that of the BCHA. - Speech perception in quiet and noise improved in the aided situation similarly for both hearing devices.

5. Conclusions

Our results suggest that ABCD is a valid treatment for patients with conductive hearing loss that cannot undergo bone conduction aid implant surgery. It is also important to consider bilateral aids in order to deal with situations in which binaural hearing is fundamental.

Author Contributions: Conceptualization: E.O. and E.M.; Methodology: E.M. and S.G.; Software: I.C.; Formal analysis: R.M.; Investigation: S.G.; Data curation: G.P.; Writing-original draft preparation: E.M., R.L., V.G.; Writing-review editing: V.G., R.L., G.R.; Supervision: E.O., E.M., G.R. All authors have read and agreed to the published version of the manuscript.

Funding: This research received no external funding.

Institutional Review Board Statement: Not applicable.

Informed Consent Statement: Informed consent was obtained from all subjects involved in the study.

Data Availability Statement: The data presented in this study are available on request from the corresponding author.

Conflicts of Interest: The authors declare no conflict of interest.

References

1. Rosenfeld, R.M.; Culpepper, L.; Doyle, K.J.; Grundfast, K.M.; Hoberman, A.; Kenna, M.A.; Lieberthal, A.S.; Mahoney, M.; Wahl, R.A.; Woods, C.R.; et al. Clinical Practice Guideline: Otitis Media with Effusion. *Otolaryngol. Neck Surg.* **2004**, *130*, S95–S118. [CrossRef] [PubMed]
2. Ebert, C.S.; Pillsbury, H.C. Otitis Media: Background and Science. In *Managing the Allergic Patient*; Elsevier: Amsterdam, The Netherlands, 2008; pp. 175–191.
3. Robb, M.P.; Psak, J.L.; Pang-Ching, G.K. Chronic otitis media and early speech development: A case study. *Int. J. Pediatr. Otorhinolaryngol.* **1993**, *26*, 117–127. [CrossRef]

4. Rach, G.H.; Zielhuis, G.A.; Broek, P.V.D. The influence of chronic persistent otitis media with effusion on language development of 2- to 4-year-olds. *Int. J. Pediatr. Otorhinolaryngol.* **1988**, *15*, 253–261. [CrossRef]
5. Boudewyns, A.; Declau, F.; Ende, J.V.D.; Van Kerschaver, E.; Dirckx, S.; Brandt, A.H.-V.D.; Van de Heyning, P. Otitis Media With Effusion. *Otol. Neurotol.* **2011**, *32*, 799–804. [CrossRef] [PubMed]
6. Cai, T.; McPherson, B. Hearing loss in children with otitis media with effusion: A systematic review. *Int. J. Audiol.* **2016**, *56*, 65–76. [CrossRef] [PubMed]
7. O'Niel, M.B.; Runge, C.L.; Friedland, D.R.; Kerschner, J.E. Patient Outcomes in Magnet-Based Implantable Auditory Assist Devices. *JAMA Otolaryngol. Neck Surg.* **2014**, *140*, 513–520. [CrossRef] [PubMed]
8. Turrini, M.; Cutugno, F.; Maturi, P.; Prosser, S.; Leoni, F.A.; Arslan, E. Bisyllabic words for speech audiometry: A new italian material. *Acta Otorhinolaryngol. Ital.* **1993**, *13*, 63–77. [PubMed]
9. Koopmans, W.J.A.; Goverts, S.T.; Smits, C. Speech Recognition Abilities in Normal-Hearing Children 4 to 12 Years of Age in Stationary and Interrupted Noise. *Ear Heart* **2018**, *39*, 1091–1103. [CrossRef] [PubMed]
10. Cai, T.; McPherson, B.; Li, C.; Yang, F. Hearing Loss in Children With Otitis Media With Effusion: Actual and Simulated Effects on Speech Perception. *Ear Heart* **2018**, *39*, 645–655. [CrossRef] [PubMed]
11. Dahm, V.; Baumgartner, W.-D.; Liepins, R.; Arnoldner, C.; Riss, D. First Results with a New, Pressure-free, Adhesive Bone Conduction Hearing Aid. *Otol. Neurotol.* **2018**, *39*, 748–754. [CrossRef] [PubMed]
12. Kuthubutheen, J.; Broadbent, C.; Marino, R.; Távora-Vieira, D. The Use of a Novel, Nonsurgical Bone Conduction Hearing Aid System for the Treatment of Conductive Hearing Loss. *Otol. Neurotol.* **2020**, *41*, 948–955. [CrossRef] [PubMed]
13. Snapp, H.; Vogt, K.; Agterberg, M.J. Bilateral bone conduction stimulation provides reliable binaural cues for localization. *Heart Res.* **2020**, *388*, 107881. [CrossRef] [PubMed]
14. Neumann, K.; Thomas, J.P.; Voelter, C.; Dazert, S. A new adhesive bone conduction hearing system effectively treats conductive hearing loss in children. *Int. J. Pediatr. Otorhinolaryngol.* **2019**, *122*, 117–125. [CrossRef] [PubMed]
15. Dahm, V.; Auinger, A.B.; Liepins, R.; Baumgartner, W.-D.; Riss, D.; Arnoldner, C. A Randomized Cross-over Trial Comparing a Pressure-free, Adhesive to a Conventional Bone Conduction Hearing Device. *Otol. Neurotol.* **2019**, *40*, 571–577. [CrossRef] [PubMed]
16. Favoreel, A.; Heuninck, E.; Mansbach, A.-L. Audiological benefit and subjective satisfaction of children with the ADHEAR audio processor and adhesive adapter. *Int. J. Pediatr. Otorhinolaryngol.* **2020**, *129*, 109729. [CrossRef] [PubMed]
17. Gawliczek, T.; Munzinger, F.; Anschuetz, L.; Caversaccio, M.; Kompis, M.; Wimmer, W. Unilateral and Bilateral Audiological Benefit With an Adhesively Attached, Noninvasive Bone Conduction Hearing System. *Otol. Neurotol.* **2018**, *39*, 1025–1030. [CrossRef] [PubMed]
18. Mertens, G.; Gilles, A.; Bouzegta, R.; Van de Heyning, P. A Prospective Randomized Crossover Study in Single Sided Deafness on the New Non-Invasive Adhesive Bone Conduction Hearing System. *Otol. Neurotol.* **2018**, *39*, 940–949. [CrossRef] [PubMed]
19. Brill, I.T.; Brill, S.; Stark, T. Neue Möglichkeiten der Rehabilitation bei Schallleitungsschwerhörigkeit. *HNO* **2019**, *67*, 698–705. [CrossRef] [PubMed]
20. Weiss, R.; Loth, A.; Leinung, M.; Balster, S.; Hirth, D.; Stöver, T.; Helbig, S.; Kramer, S. A new adhesive bone conduction hearing system as a treatment option for transient hearing loss after middle ear surgery. *Eur. Arch. Oto-Rhino-Laryngol.* **2019**, *277*, 751–759. [CrossRef] [PubMed]
21. Almuhawas, F.; Alzhrani, F.; Saleh, S.; AlSanosi, A.; Yousef, M. Auditory Performance and Subjective Satisfaction with the ADHEAR System. *Audiol. Neurotol.* **2021**, *26*, 1–10. [CrossRef] [PubMed]

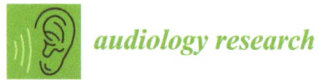

Review

Sound Localization and Lateralization by Bilateral Bone Conduction Devices, Middle Ear Implants, and Cartilage Conduction Hearing Aids

Kimio Shiraishi

Department of Communication Design Science, Faculty of Design, Kyushu University, Fukuoka 815-0032, Japan; shiraishi.kimio.356@m.kyushu-u.ac.jp; Tel.: +81-92-804-8657

Abstract: Sound localization in daily life is one of the important functions of binaural hearing. Bilateral bone conduction devices (BCDs), middle ear implants, and cartilage conduction hearing aids have been often applied for patients with conductive hearing loss (CHL) or mixed hearing loss, for example, resulting from bilateral microtia and aural atresia. In this review, factors affecting the accuracy of sound localization with bilateral BCDs, middle ear implants, and cartilage conduction hearing aids were classified into four categories: (1) types of device, (2) experimental conditions, (3) participants, and (4) pathways from the stimulus sound to both cochleae. Recent studies within the past 10 years on sound localization and lateralization by BCDs, middle ear implants, and cartilage conduction hearing aids were discussed. Most studies showed benefits for sound localization or lateralization with bilateral devices. However, the judgment accuracy was generally lower than that for normal hearing, and the localization errors tended to be larger than for normal hearing. Moreover, it should be noted that the degree of accuracy in sound localization by bilateral BCDs varied considerably among patients. Further research on sound localization is necessary to analyze the complicated mechanism of bone conduction, including suprathreshold air conduction with bilateral devices.

Keywords: localization; lateralization; binaural hearing; hearing loss; bone conduction device; middle ear implant; cartilage conduction hearing aid

1. Introduction

We are surrounded by many different sounds and we can easily know where they are and how far they are from us. This ability is called "localization". According to Moore [1], the term "localization" refers to determining the direction and distance of a sound source. It is well known that sound localization in the horizontal plane is mediated by two cues: interaural time difference (ITD) and interaural level difference (ILD). The ITD is defined as the difference in arrival time between the two ears and is the most important cue to sound localization for low-frequency components [2]. The ILD is defined as the difference in the level of a sound at the two ears caused mainly by the head "shadowing" effect for high-frequency components [2]. Sound localization in the vertical plane is accomplished through filtering by the pinnae and the head itself. This filtering can be expressed in "head-related transfer functions (HRTFs)" [1]. The HRTF changes in the vertical and horizontal planes depending on the angle of incidence of the sound. So, with regard to hearing aids, there are differences in the HRTF depending on the angle at which the sound is presented from the loudspeaker when the device is worn, or where the device microphone is placed on the head. Related to sound localization, the term "lateralization" is used to describe the apparent location of the sound source within the head, when the stimulus is presented via headphones or bone vibrators. Sometimes the term "lateralization" is also used to judge whether the sound appears from the right or the left when presented by a loudspeaker [3].

Hearing loss affects sound localization and causes serious problems in daily life for the hearing-impaired. Häusler et al. (1983) [4] investigated the localization ability of persons with different types of hearing loss, such as conductive hearing loss (CHL), bilateral or unilateral sensorineural hearing losses, unilateral dead ear, and central hearing loss. For example, the localization ability in CHL is close to normal hearing if the loss does not exceed 25 dB HL. However, both unilateral and bilateral hearing losses greater than 35 dB HL affect the localization ability of both horizontal and vertical angle discrimination. Kramer et al. (1995, 1998) [5,6] investigated the extent to which individuals see themselves as being handicapped by gathering self-reports of 239 hearing-impaired persons with varying types of hearing loss. They showed that problems with sound intelligibility under noise and, indeed, auditory localization were considered as the most frequent disabilities.

The usefulness of bone conduction devices (BCDs) to assist persons with CHL, such as bone conduction hearing aids (BCHAs), was already pointed out in the early 1950s [7]. For a long time, unilateral fitting of BCHAs was commonly applied, even for persons with bilateral CHL caused by microtia, aural atresia, and chronic otitis media. One reason for the unilateral application is that the transcranial attenuation (TA) of bone conduction (BC) sound by a BCD is very small (10 dB), so it will stimulate both cochleae to almost the same extent [8]. In 1977, a percutaneous bone-anchored hearing aid (BAHA) was developed that avoids most of the drawbacks of conventional BCHAs [9,10]. Snik et al. (1998) [8] reported that sound localization, as indicated by the percentage of correct identification (within 45°), improved by 53% with binaural listening for three patients with BAHA(s) that were unilaterally or bilaterally fitted. Following this, significant improvement in sound localization with bilateral BAHAs has further been reported by Bosman et al. (2001) [3] and Priwin et al. (2004) [11]. In a systematic review of the literature from 1977 to 2011 by Janssen et al. (2012) [12], comparisons were made between unilateral and bilateral BCD(s) in participants with bilateral CHL or mixed hearing loss. The authors stated that the bilateral BAHA condition was shown to improve localization and lateralization, although it was difficult to appreciate the magnitude of this effect, given that only Priwin et al. (2007) [13] compared performances between hearing-impaired persons and a normal-hearing control group.

For bone-conducted sound lateralization, Kaga et al. (2001) [14] found, using a self-recording apparatus that measured ITD and ILD, that the abilities were maintained in many patients with bilateral microtia and aural atresia. Schmerber et al. (2005) [15] obtained time-intensity trading functions using ITD and ILD in the same ear from patients with bilateral congenital aural atresia, and showed that time-intensity trading was present in the patients. They concluded that a binaural fitting of BCHAs might optimize binaural hearing and improve sound lateralization, and recommended systematic bilateral fitting in aural atresia patients.

Further advances in technology have led to the development of various kinds of BCDs apart from conventional BCHAs with a steel-spring headband or with framed glasses. Reinfeldt et al. (2015) [16] categorized these as conventional skin-drive BCDs, passive transcutaneous skin-drive BCDs, percutaneous direct-drive BCDs, and active transcutaneous direct-drive BCDs. Recently, a non-surgical adhesive BCD has been made commercially available as well [17]. Moreover, cartilage conduction hearing aids (CCHAs) have been developed by Hosoi et al. (2010) [18], without the strong pressure of the steel spring as used in conventional BCHAs or surgical operations for BAHAs.

So far, research on sound localization thus has been carried out using the various kinds of devices mentioned above. Most of the studies have reported that bilaterally fitted devices showed more improved sound localization than the unilaterally fitted ones. As the basis, Zeitooni et al. (2016) [19] investigated the effects of binaural hearing with bilateral BCHAs, measuring the spatial release from masking, the binaural intelligibility level difference, the binaural masking level difference, and the precedence effect in adults with normal hearing. In all tests, the results with bilateral BC stimulation at the BCHA position illustrated an ability to extract binaural cues similar to BC stimulation at the mastoid position. They, however, did not test sound localization, the accuracy of which can be affected by various factors, such as the type of device, the participants, and the experimental method.

The present review aimed to discuss the factors affecting sound localization or lateralization, as well as their accuracy, for persons with bilateral (simulated) CHL using bilateral devices. For the first aim, the factors affecting sound localization and lateralization were classified, and the relevant research is discussed. For the second aim, regarding the accuracy of sound localization and lateralization using a multi-loudspeaker system, rather than a questionnaire such as "The Speech, Spatial and Qualities of Hearing Scale (SSQ) [20], the clinical literature related to persons with hearing loss or normal hearing was searched on "Google Scholar". The keywords for this search were "bone conduction", "localization", "bilateral", and "conductive hearing loss" for sound localization, and "bone conduction", "lateralization", "bilateral", and "conductive hearing loss" for sound lateralization. The search was performed for literature from 2012 to August 2021 because Janssen et al. (2012) [12] had already reviewed the literature from 1977 to 2011. The strategy used to select the literature for the second aim was as follows.

First, the keyword search conditions in "Google Scholar" were set to exclude "Include patents" and "Include quotes". The search resulted in 1079 hits for sound localization and 670 hits for sound lateralization. These contents were sorted in descending order of relevance. The 1000 hits of the upper limit displayed from the top for sound localization and the 670 hits for sound lateralization were investigated. After inspection of the URLs, it was found that 982 hits for sound localization and 653 hits for sound lateralization were valid for analysis, after excluding links that displayed a "Not found" or "Not connected" message. These hit numbers were set as the initial values for screening for this review. The screening process and the number of resulting hits are shown in Figure 1. As a result, nine scientific articles for the review of sound localization and five for sound lateralization were picked up. The five articles for sound lateralization, however, were the same as the nine articles for localization, so these nine articles were selected. Furthermore, the nine articles for sound localization were categorized into those with normal-hearing participants with bilateral simulated CHL (three articles: Table 1) and those with bilateral CHL (six articles: Table 2).

Table 1. Studies on sound localization or lateralization with bone conduction for simulated conductive hearing loss from 2012 to August 2021.

No.	Authors (Year)	Participants	Devices	Stimuli	Presentation Levels	Setup	Test Conditions
1	Gawliczek et al. (2018a) [21]	15 participants with induced bilateral CHL	aBCD(s) (ADHEAR) and BCD(s) attached to a softband (Baha5)	White noise (200 ms duration)	Between 60 and 65 dB SPL	Twelve loudspeakers (aligned in a horizontal circular set up: an angular interval of 30°)	Evaluation of BCD1 (ADHEAR), comparison between unilateral and bilateral fitting, and comparison between BCD1 and BCD2 (Baha 5)
2	Gawliczek et al. (2018b) [22]	15 participants with simulated bilateral CHL with a combination of ear plugs and silicon mould material	BCD(s) (Baha5) (SoundArc and a softband)	White noise (200 ms duration)	60, 65, and 70 dB SPL	Twelve loudspeakers (aligned in a horizontal circular set up: an angular interval of 30°)	(i) Unaided, (ii) aided with one BAHS sound processor mounted on a SoundArc, (iii) aided with 2 BAHS sound processors on a single SoundArc, (iv) aided with one BAHS sound processor on a softband, and (v) aided with 2 BAHS sound processors on a single soft band
3	Snapp et al. (2020) [23]	11 listeners with simulated CHL with plug(s)	aBCD(s) (ADHER)	Broadband (BB; 0.5–20 kHz), high-pass (HP; 3–20 kHz), and low-pass (LP; 0.5–1.5 kHz) noise bursts (150 ms duration)	45, 55, and 65 dB A	Twenty-four loudspeakers (the horizontal (±70°) and vertical (+40°/−30°) planes (The speakers were covered by a black, sound emitting curtain)	Normal hearing, unilateral plug, unilateral plug + ipsilateral aBCD, unilateral plug + ipsilateral aBCD+ contralateral pinna mold, bilateral plugs, bilateral plugs + bilateral aBCDs, and bilateral plugs + unilateral aBCD

Abbreviations: aBCD, adhesive bone conduction device; BAHS, bone-anchored hearing systems; CHL, conductive hearing loss.

Table 2. Studies on sound localization or lateralization with bone conduction device(s) for bilateral conductive hearing loss from 2012 to August 2021.

No.	Authors (Year)	Participants	Devices	Stimuli	Presentation Levels	Setup	Test Conditions
1	Dun et al. (2013) [24]	10 children with severe bilateral CHL due to congenital major or minor ear anomalies with microtia or anotia or due to resistant chronic inflammation	Unilateral (right or left) BCD and bilateral BCDs (Baha)	Broadband noise; (0.5 to 20 kHz, 500 ms duration)	Randomly in 10 dB steps within the 40 to 70 dB SPL range	MAA: two loudspeakers ($\pm 90°$, $\pm 60°$, $\pm 30°$, $\pm 15°$, $\pm 10°$, and $\pm 5°$)	Unilateral condition (right or left) and bilateral condition
2	Fan et al. (2020) [25]	32 patients with congenital bilateral microtia-atresia	Bilateral BCDs (BB and 1 ADHEAR)	White noise	65, 70, and 75 dB SPL	Seven loudspeakers (30° interval from $-90°$ to $+90°$)	Three conditions: unaided, unilateral BCD (BB) and bilateral BCDs (BB plus contralateral ADHEAR)
3	Besten et al. (2020) [26]	10 children with congenital bilateral CHL, and 1 child with acquired bilateral CHL	One or two percutaneous BCDs (Baha Divino, Baha BP100, or Baha4)	MAA: a broadband noise burst (bandwidth 0.5–20 kHz, 500 ms duration) Sound localization: broadband noise bursts (bandwidth 0.5–8 kHz, 150 ms duration)	MAA: 55, 60 or 65 dB SPL Sound localization: 50, 60, or 70 dB SPL	MAA: two loudspeakers ($\pm 90°$, $\pm 60°$, $\pm 30°$, $\pm 15°$, $\pm 10°$, and $\pm 5°$). Sound localization: $-75°$ (left) to $+75°$ (right).	Unilateral BCD on the left side, unilateral BCD on the right side, and bilateral BCDs
4	Nishimura et al. (2020) [27]	13 patients with bilateral aural atresia	CC hearing aids	Pink noise (500 ms duration including a rise/fall time of 50 ms)	65 dB SPL	Eight loudspeakers (full circle at 45° interval)	Unaided, aided with previously used hearing aids (air conduction or BC hearing aids), and aided with CC hearing aids
5	Ren et al. (2021) [28]	12 children with mild-to-severe bilateral conductive hearing loss due to congenital microtia	Unilateral or Bilateral BCD(s) (ADHEAR)	A recorded gunshot sound	65 dB SPL	Twelve loudspeakers (a semi-circle, ranging from $-82.5°$ to $82.5°$ with 15° intervals	Unaided, unilateral aided and bilateral aided
6	Caspers et al. (2021) [29]	15 adults with bilateral CHL and mixed HL (congenital and acquired HL)	Percutaneous BCDs (Baha4 or Baha5)	Broadband noise (BB; 0.5 to 20 kHz), high-pass (HP; 3–20 kHz) and low-pass (LP; 0.5–1.5 kHz)	45, 55, and 65 dB SPL for BB stimuli; and 55 dB SPL for HL and LP stimuli	Twenty-four loudspeakers positioned on an arc between $+70°$ (right) and $-70°$ (left) azimuth and between $+40°$ (up) and $-30°$ (down)	Unilateral aided conditions (right and left) and bilateral aided condition

Abbreviations: BCD, bone conduction device; BB, bonebridge; CHL, conductive hearing loss; CC, cartilage conduction; HL, hearing loss; MAA, minimum audible angle.

Initial values were set at N=982 for sound localization and n=653 for sound lateralization, respectively.

1. Is it a "journal article" written in English with a full text, not a "review", "conference paper", "case report", "thesis", or "book" from 2012 to August 2021?
   Yes (N=421, n=292), No (N=561, n=361).

2. Does the article use "bone conduction" and "(sound) localization" or "lateralization" in the title, the abstract, or keywords?
   Yes (N=59, n=35), No (N=362, n=257).

3. Do the participants have "bilateral (simulated) conductive hearing loss or mixed hearing loss", rather than "unilateral conductive hearing loss", "sensorineural hearing loss", or "single-sided deafness"?
   Yes (N=14, n=8), No (N=45, n=27).

4. Do the participants use bilateral bone (cartilage) conduction devices or middle ear implants rather than air conduction hearing aids?
   Yes (N=11, n=6), No (N=3, n=2).

5. Does the research described in the article employ a "multi-loudspeaker system" to measure sound localization or lateralization ability?
   Yes (N=9, n=5), No (N=2, n=1).

Figure 1. Screening process and the number of resulting hits regarding the literature about the accuracy of sound localization and lateralization using a multi-loudspeaker system (2012 to August 2021). "N=" and "n=" represent the hit number for "localization" and "lateralization", respectively.

2. Factors Affecting the Accuracy of Sound Localization or Lateralization

Figure 2 schematically shows the factors that affect the accuracy of sound localization or lateralization of bone-conducted sound for a patient with bilateral CHL. These factors were roughly classified into four categories: (1) devices, (2) experimental conditions, (3) participants, and (4) pathways from the stimulus sound to both cochleae. Tables 1 and 2 show the studies on sound localization or lateralization with details about the authors (year), devices, stimuli, presentation levels, setup, and test conditions for normal-hearing participants with simulated CHL and participants with bilateral CHL, respectively, in chronological order.

2.1. Devices

A conventional skin-drive BCHA that vibrates the bone via the skin consists of a microphone, an amplifier, and a BC transducer (vibrator or actuator) with a soft headband (softband), a steel spring headband, or spectacles [16]. The conventional electromagnetic bone transducers have a frequency curve that falls off below 0.25 kHz and above 4 kHz, with a resonance peak at 0.2–0.6 kHz [30]. This limited frequency range may affect the accuracy of front–back sound localization, because front–back localization appears to be coded in the energy contained within the 3–7 kHz bandwidth of a signal [31]. A giant magnetostrictive BC transducer with a frequency range from 0.5–30 kHz developed by Sakai et al. (2016) [30] may be useful for sound localization experiments. In addition, for bilaterally fitted BCDs, both the microphones and transducers are located a few centimeters apart in order to reduce acoustic feedback. Thus, the ITD and ILD are slightly affected depending on the position of the BCD's microphones.

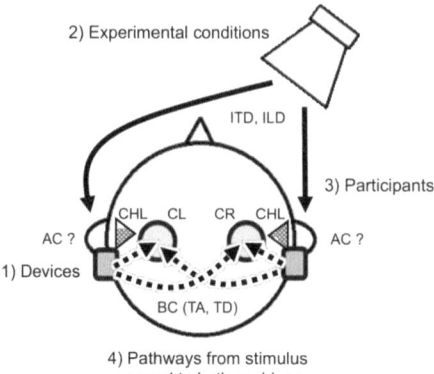

Figure 2. Factors affecting the accuracy of sound localization or lateralization of bone-conducted sound for a participant with (simulated) bilateral conductive hearing loss. Abbreviations: AC, air conduction; BC, bone conduction; CHL, conductive hearing loss; CL, left cochlea; CR, right cochlea; ITD, interaural time difference; ILD, interaural level difference; TA, transcranial attenuation; TD, transcranial delay.

The principles and characteristics of the BCDs shown in Tables 1 and 2 are, in brief, the following. Gawlizek et al. (2018a) [21] studied sound localization using two kinds of passive transcutaneous skin-drive BCDs. One BCD was the ADHEAR device (MED-EL, Innsbruck, Austria), where the transducer is glue-attached without pressure using an acrylic plate. The ADHEARs were also applied bilaterally by Ren et al. (2021) [28]. The audio frequency range is from 0.25 kHz to 8 kHz and signal processing occurs with automatic adaptive directional microphones (DMs) [32]. The other BCD is the Baha5 with a softband (Cochlear Inc., Mölnlycke, Sweden), which has an almost similar audio frequency range (Baha Connect: 0.25–7 kHz; Baha Attract: 0.25–6.3 kHz) [33]. Moreover, this device has a function of "Active Balanced Directionality", controlled by the Scene Classifier, which gives wearers the ability to seamlessly blend between omnidirectional and directional settings [34]. The Bonebridge (BB) (MED-EL, Innsbruck, Austria), an active transcutaneous device, is a semi-implantable system consisting of an implantable part and an externally worn audio processor. The audio frequency range is from 0.25 kHz to 8 kHz and signal processing occurs with DM [35]. In CCHAs (HB-J1CC, Rion, Tokyo, Japan), the sound is delivered to the aural cartilage using a small and lightweight transducer that is attached to the aural cartilage without high-contact pressure. In contrast to the conventional BCHA, the transducer is placed without a headband, which is more comfortable for wearing, with better aesthetics. Surgery is not required with CCHAs, unlike with BAHAs and other middle ear implants [27]. The acoustical output of the transducer measured with the artificial mastoid has a mountain-shaped frequency response with a peak at 0.8–2 kHz [18]. The sound pressure levels in the external canal show double peaks at approximately 0.8 kHz and 2.5 kHz [36]. Nishimura et al. (2020) [27] used the device to study sound localization for the first time.

In studies on sound localization, various kinds of devices have been used for (simulated) CHL. The devices differ in microphone type and position, transducer positions, and signal processing. These differences may affect the accuracy of sound localization. Denk et al. (2019) [37] investigated the impacts of the microphone's location, the signal bandwidth, and different equalization approaches, and showed that the microphone's location was the governing factor for localization abilities with linear hearing devices. Regarding the relationship between adaptive DMs and localization in hearing aids, both the studies by Keidser et al. (2006) [38] and Van den Bogaert et al. (2006) [39] showed that independently operating adaptive DMs have an adverse effect on scores in a laboratory experiment. For synchronized adaptive DMs, the results are inconsistent. Namely,

Keidser et al. (2006) [38] reported no benefit, while Ibrahim et al. (2013) [40] showed improvements for some stimuli. Johnson et al. (2017) [41] described that the difference between premium-feature hearing aids (i.e., with multi-channel adaptive DMs, pinna effect simulation, and an advanced synchronization function) and basic-feature hearing aids (i.e., with single-channel adaptive DMs and a basic synchronization function) was not significant in self-reported everyday sound localization. Caspers et al. (2021) [29] switched off adaptive DM and noise reduction in the setting of BCDs to avoid deterioration in localization performance.

Regarding the stimulation position of the bone-conducted sound, Stenfelt (2012) [42] reported that the median transcranial attenuation (TA) is 2 to 3 dB lower than at the mastoid when measured at the BCHA position. Dobrev et al. (2016) [43] investigated the influence of stimulus position on BC hearing sensitivity with a BC transducer attached using a headband. They concluded that stimulation on a position superior-anterior to the pinna provides more efficient BC transmission than stimulation on the mastoid. Moreover, the contact condition of the actuator at the stimulation position affects sound localization. Asakura et al. (2019) [44] reported that bone-conducted binaural sound localization performance could increase, depending on the contact force and the position of the actuator device.

2.2. Experimental Conditions

2.2.1. Measurement Methods

When sound is presented by a loudspeaker in a sound field, two methods can be mainly used to measure the ability of sound localization. One is to identify one loudspeaker's direction from multiple loudspeakers arranged in a semicircular or circular way relative to the participant. When multiple loudspeakers are arranged in a circle (e.g., see No. 1 and No. 2 in Table 1 and No. 4 in Table 2), it is easy to create front/back confusions, in that a stimulus in front of the participant is localized to the rear or vice versa [45]. The frequency of front/back confusions tends to increase as the bandwidth of the stimulus is decreased [46]. Front/back confusion is caused by the difficulty of localization using the ITD and the ILD in the experimental room, although moving one's head or experience from the surrounding sound environment can help to localize a sound source in daily life. The second method is to discriminate the minimum audible angle (MAA), which is defined as the smallest detectable difference between the azimuths of two identical sounds [47]. In this method, immediately after presenting the reference sound, the sound source's position is shifted to the left or right, and the MAA is measured by asking the participant to answer whether the test sound is heard from the left or right of the reference. Already in 1958, Mills [47] described that the MAA for a tone of 1 kHz or higher is about 1 degree at an azimuth of 0 degrees. The discrimination task is also easy for children to measure the ultimate sensitivity of the localization system [4]. For example, Lovett et al. (2012) [48] reported that children showed adult levels of performance from age 3 years for left–right discrimination, and from age 6 years for localization. Asp et al. (2016) [49] developed a corneal reflection eye-tracking technique to record pupil positions toward spatially distributed continuous auditory and visual stimuli to assess horizontal sound localization accuracy from 6 months of age. They showed that the method provides an objective and fast assessment of horizontal sound localization accuracy.

2.2.2. Stimulus Conditions

Pink noise, white noise, and broadband noise are often used as the stimulus sound, as shown in Tables 1 and 2. When used with wideband frequency, it is necessary to confirm whether the stimulus sound is sufficiently reproduced in the device's frequency range. Yost et al. (2014) [50] described that the accuracy of sound source localization increases as the bandwidth of the stimulus sound increases, and that stimuli with a wide range of one octave or more have the best sound source localization accuracy. The onset duration of the stimulus also affects sound source localization [51]. Stimulus levels are often used at a level of 65 dB SPL or 65 dB A, as shown in Tables 1 and 2, which corresponds to the intensity level of conversation. When the stimulus presentation level becomes larger, it exceeds the earplugged air conduction threshold or the actual patient's threshold with CHL. In this case, both the bone-conducted sound, via bilaterally fitted BCDs, and the suprathreshold air-conducted sound may be presented simultaneously to the cochleae and interfere with the sound localization cues (Figure 2).

2.3. Participants

There are merits and demerits in sound localization experiments for employing, respectively, participants with normal hearing (bilateral simulated CHL) and patients with bilateral CHL.

2.3.1. Normal-Hearing Participants with Simulated CHL

Normal-hearing participants are used to simulate bilateral CHL by blocking their ears with earplugs (and earmuffs) or earmolds. Normal-hearing participants with simulated CHL have the advantages of normally developed hearing, and the BC thresholds of the left and right ears under masking can be accurately measured. The participants thus can be assumed to be a homogeneous study group. However, there is a limit of sound insulation by earplugs and earmuffs, and the audiogram of simulated CHL depends on the sound insulation performance. For example, in an experiment to investigate the effect of simulated unilateral hearing loss on horizontal sound localization by Asp et al. (2018) [52], the degrees of hearing loss were mild hearing loss (average threshold of 30 dB HL across 0.5, 1, 2, and 4 kHz) with an earplug, and moderate hearing loss (average threshold of 43 dB HL across 0.5, 1, 2, and 4 kHz) with an earplug and earmuff. Furthermore, both audiogram configurations showed larger hearing loss in the high frequencies than in the low frequencies. Compared with actual patients with CHL, these degrees of simulated hearing loss and the audiogram configuration may differ substantially.

2.3.2. Patients with Bilateral CHL

For patients with bilateral CHL, it is clinically meaningful to examine their sound localization ability. The heterogeneity of the study group with respect to the duration of deafness, the degree of hearing loss, the symmetry of hearing, and the period of device use makes it difficult to generalize the results. Furthermore, there are few reports on how localization accuracy is affected by whether the CHL is congenital or acquired. In the case of congenital aural atresia and microtia, the auditory system may not always be fully developed for both ears. Kaga et al. (2016) [53] carried out a sound lateralization test (ILD and ITD) in 18 patients with unilateral microtia and atresia, after reconstruction of the auricle and external canal and fitting a canal-type hearing aid for the operated ear. Their results showed that the ability to discriminate the ILD was acquired in all of the patients, whereas that to discriminate ITD was acquired in only half of the patients. They stated that the difference must be caused by late-development brain plasticity for binaural hearing. Caspers et al. (2021) [29] reported that bilaterally fitted patients with bilaterally acquired hearing loss, as well as patients with congenital hearing loss, were capable of localizing sounds (quite) accurately. For the obtained bilateral BC thresholds, they described that sound lateralization was more accurate in patients with symmetric and near-normal BC thresholds when compared with patients with either asymmetric BC thresholds or patients with BC thresholds of 25 dB and higher, and that normal symmetric thresholds did not warrant good localization. Here, when the degree of CHL in both ears became larger in a patient with bilateral CHL, it was difficult to obtain an actual BC threshold due to over-masking (the so-called "masking dilemma") [54].

When the participants are children, their ages can affect the ability of sound localization. From measurement of ITD and ILD with a self-recording apparatus, Kaga (1992) [55] showed that the ability to localize sound sources rapidly developed between the ages of 5 and 6 years. In addition, for children with bilateral congenital microtia, Ren et al. (2021) [28] reported that the improvement in sound localization was also negatively related to the malformation degree of the patient's head. Apart from this, the ability of sound localization can improve with training. Following tests with 11 participants with unilateral severe to profound hearing loss, Firszt et al. (2015) [56] reported that the eight participants with the poorest localization ability improved significantly following training, while the three participants with the best pre-training ability showed the least training benefit. Taking all the abovementioned factors into consideration, in experiments with patients, it is generally difficult to have a group with the same patient background.

2.4. Pathways from the Sound Source to the Cochleae

Sound localization by binaural hearing with devices is mainly mediated by two pathways: (1) the pathways from the sound source to the microphones of the bilateral devices, and (2) the pathways from the bone-conducted sound induced by both devices to both cochleae (Figure 2).

2.4.1. Pathways from the Sound Source to the Microphones of the Bilateral Devices

The ITD detection threshold varies depending on the type of sound (e.g., the use of a band-limited random noise from 0.15–1.7 kHz, a 1 kHz tone, or a 1-millisecond click) and ranges from 9 to 28 µs [57]. ITD reaches its maximum when the sound arrives from the side, and its value is then about 650 µs [2]. The detection threshold of ILD is about 1 to 2 dB [2].

2.4.2. Pathways from Bone-Conducted Sound induced by Devices to the Cochleae

It is generally accepted that bone-conducted sound transmission in the human skull is linear, at least for frequencies between 0.1 and 10 kHz and up to 77 dB HL [58]. However, the relationship between the mechanism of bone-conducted sound propagation within the skull and BC hearing has not yet been fully elucidated. Eeg-Olofsson (2012) [58] reported that the main components that contribute to BC hearing are: the occlusion effect, middle ear ossicle inertia, inner ear fluid inertia, compression and expansion of the cochlea, and the cerebrospinal fluid pathway. When both devices stimulate the left and right cochleae, an ILD by the TA and an ITD by the transcranial delay (TD) between the ipsilateral and the contralateral cochleae to the stimulation may assist sound localization.

- Transcranial attenuation (TA):

Stenfelt et al. (2012) [42] studied TA in 28 cases of unilateral deafness using four stimulus positions (ipsilateral, contralateral mastoid, ipsilateral, and contralateral position) for a BCHA at 31 frequencies from 0.25 to 8 kHz. The results showed that with stimulation at the mastoid, the median TA was 3 dB to 5 dB at frequencies up to 0.5 kHz and close to 0 dB between 0.5 to 1.8 kHz. The TA was close to 10 dB at 3 to 5 kHz, and became slightly less at the highest frequencies measured (4 dB at 8 kHz). Furthermore, the intersubjective variability was large for each frequency (around 40 dB), but there were small differences in the general trends of TA between individuals. For normal-hearing participants, Stenfelt et al. (2013) [59] reported that the TA showed almost the same tendencies as in participants with unilateral deafness. Recently, Röösli et al. (2021) [60] reported that TA is affected by stimulus location, the coupling of the bone conduction hearing aid to the underlying tissue, and the properties of the head (such as the geometry of the head, thickness of the skin and/or skull, changes due to aging, iatrogenic changes such as bone removal during mastoidectomy, and occlusion of the external auditory canal).

- Transcranial delay (TD):

TD between the ipsilateral and contralateral cochleae with stimulation by a BCD on one side is related to the propagation velocity of bone-conducted sound in the skull. Franke (1956) [61] placed two pickups on the frontal and parietal regions of a human skull and observed the BC velocity as the difference in the waveform between the two pickups when stimulating the forehead. As a result, the propagation velocity increased from low frequencies to high frequencies: it was about 150 m/s near frequencies of 0.5 kHz and about 300 m/s at frequencies above 1.5 kHz, which then almost remained constant. Wigand et al. (1964) [62], however, reported that the BC velocity of the skull base is 3000 m/s. Contrary to this, by using a psychophysical method, Tonndorf et al. (1981) [63] measured the propagation velocity of bone-conducted sound and reported that indeed it was about 55 m/s near frequencies of 0.5–0.75 kHz and about 330 m/s at frequencies above 2 kHz for the human skull. By measuring the mechanical point impedance from 27 positions on the skull surface in six intact cadaver heads, Stenfelt and Goode (2005) [64] reported that the phase velocity in the cranial bone is estimated to increase from around 250 m/s at 2 kHz to 300 m/s at 10 kHz. Although the propagation velocity value in the skull thus differs depending on the frequency of the bone-conducted sound, the object (dry skull, living subject, human cadaver), and the measurement method, this velocity indicates the TD of the bone-conducted sound for ipsilateral mastoid stimulation between the ipsilateral and the contralateral cochleae. Zeitooni et al. (2016) [19] described that the TD between the cochleae for mastoid placement of BC stimulation is estimated to be 0.3 to 0.5 ms at frequencies above 1 kHz, while there are no reliable estimates at lower frequencies.

As described above, the bone-conducted sound induced via bilateral devices can cause complicated interference for the bilateral cochleae due to TA and TD. Farrel et al. (2017) [65] measured ITD and ILD from the intracochlear pressures and stapes velocity conveyed by bilateral BC systems. They showed that the variation of the ITDs and ILDs conveyed by bone-anchored hearing devices systematically modulated cochlear inputs. They concluded that binaural disparities potentiate binaural benefit, providing a basis for improved sound localization. At the same time, transcranial cross-talk could lead to complex interactions that depend on cue type and stimulus frequency.

3. Accuracy of Sound Localization and Lateralization Using Device(s)

As mentioned above, previous studies have shown that sound localization by bone-conducted sound with bilaterally fitted devices involves a greater variety of factors than sound localization by air-conducted sound. Next, a review was made to assess how much the accuracy of sound localization by bilaterally fitted devices differs from that with unilaterally fitted devices or unaided conditions for participants with bilateral (simulated) CHL and with normal hearing. The methodology of the studies is shown in Tables 1 and 2.

3.1. Normal-Hearing Participants with Simulated CHL

Gawliczek et al. (2018a) [21] evaluated sound localization ability using two non-invasive BCDs (BCD1: ADHEAR; BCD2: Baha5 with softband) for unilateral and bilateral simulated CHL with earplugs. The mean absolute localization error (MAE) in the bilateral fitting condition improved by 34.2° for BCD1 and by 27.9° for BCD2 as compared with the unilateral fitting condition, thus resulting in a slight difference of about 7° between BCD1 and BCD2. The authors stated that the difference was caused by the ILD and ITD from different microphone positions between the BCDs. Gawliczek et al. (2018b) [22] further measured the audiological benefit of the Baha SoundArc and compared it with the known softband options. No statistically significant difference was found between the SoundArc and the softband options in any of the tests (soundfield thresholds, speech understanding in quiet and in noise, and sound localization). Using two sound processors rather than one improved the sound localization error by 5°, from 23° to 28°.

Snapp et al. (2020) [23] investigated the unilaterally and bilaterally aided benefits of aBCDs (ADHER) in normal-hearing listeners under simulated (plugged) unilateral and bilateral CHL conditions using measures of sound localization. In the listening conditions with bilateral plugs and bilateral aBCD, listeners could localize the stimuli with a high degree of accuracy. The response gains reached that of normal hearing performance for all levels, although the target response plots indicated a larger scatter and a worse MAE than in normal hearing conditions. The results for the unilateral application of the aBCD condition with bilateral plugs, however, showed a clear localization bias towards the aBCD side.

3.2. Patients with Bilateral CHL

Fan et al. (2020) [25] compared the effects of one BCD (BB) and bilateral BCDs (BB plus contralateral ADHEAR) on sound localization abilities in patients with bilateral microtia–atresia. The results showed that the response accuracy was significantly better with bilateral BCDs (22%) than with unilateral BCDs (16%). However, the percentage with bilateral BCDs did not reach the level of the unaided condition. The bias angles following unilateral and bilateral BCDs were 34.1° and 26.4°, respectively, indicating ipsilateral bias directed to the side of BB implantation. The authors stated that these findings may be explained by the partial re-establishment of ITDs and ILDs by bilateral BCDs. With regard to this partial re-establishment, they considered that the BB might have provided a relatively stronger stimulation of both cochleae compared with the contralateral ADHEAR. Ren et al. (2021) [28] also used ADHEARs bilaterally for 12 children with mild to severe bilateral CHL due to congenital microtia. They stated that unilateral fitting of ADHEAR did not improve the sound localization ability, while bilateral fitting demonstrated instant improvement in half of the patients, in that the root mean square error (RMSE) decreased from $67.9 \pm 10.9°$ (unaided condition) to $33.7 \pm 4.9°$ (bilateral fitting). For the other half of the patients, however, no significant difference was found in the RMSE between the unaided condition of $49.7 \pm 15.0°$ and the bilateral fitting of $57.7 \pm 15.1°$. Thus, they showed that the improvement in sound localization ability under bilateral fitting strongly correlated with the unaided sound localization ability: patients who perform worse when unaided tend to benefit more.

Caspers et al. (2021) [29] investigated sound localization in 15 patients bilaterally fitted with BCDs (Baha4 or Baha5) and explored clinical methods to improve localization accuracy. Sound localization was measured at baseline, and settings to optimize sound localization were added to the BCDs. At 1 month, sound localization was assessed again and localization was practiced with a series of sounds with visual feedback. At 3 months, localization performance, device use, and questionnaire scores were determined again. As a result, at baseline, one patient with congenital hearing loss demonstrated near excellent localization performance, and four other patients (three with congenital hearing loss) localized sounds (quite) accurately. Seven patients with acquired hearing loss were able to lateralize sounds (i.e., identify whether the sounds were coming from the left or right side) but could not localize sounds accurately. Three patients (one with congenital hearing loss), however, could not lateralize sounds correctly. Nevertheless, the authors concluded that the majority of experienced bilateral BCD users could lateralize sounds and one-third were able to localize sounds (quite) accurately, with robust performance over time.

Dun et al. (2013) [24] investigated whether children with bilateral CHL benefitted from their second device (i.e., the bilateral BCD (Baha)). Spatial resolution was tested with MAA in the bilateral and monaural listening conditions. The MAA decreased from 57° in the best monaural condition to 13° in the bilateral condition, thus demonstrating the advantage of bilateral BCD fitting in children with bilateral CHL. In a related study, Besten et al. (2020) [26] characterized the lateralization (MAA) of sounds and localization of sounds in children with bilateral CHL when listening with either one or two percutaneous BCDs (Baha Divino, Baha BP100, or Baha4). For lateralization of sound, in seven out of the 10 children, the MAA was 90° in one or both of the unilateral conditions, and equal to or less than 15° in the bilateral condition. The result of lateralization in the bilateral BCD condition was close to normal in nearly all the children. Sound localization thus was better with bilateral BCDs than in the unilaterally aided conditions. However, most children showed a bimodal response pattern, reflecting sound lateralization and not sound localization in the sound localization test.

Nishimura et al. (2020) [27] evaluated sound localization for patients with bilateral aural atresia using CCHAs in three conditions: unaided, aided with previously used hearing aids (air conduction HAs or BCHAs), and aided with CCHAs. The ability to distinguish sounds originating from left or right for participants aided with CCHAs was significantly better than that for other conditions. Compared with that in patients aided with previously used aids, no difference in front-back misidentification was found. The percent correct rates of 0.88 for left and 0.9 for right sound localization by CCHAs showed statistically significant improvements compared with the percent correct rates of 0.77 (left) and 0.64 (right) obtained with previously used HAs. The authors hypothesized that the reason might be the contribution of vibration sensation due to lower contact pressure by the transducer of CCHAs in comparison with conventional BCHAs.

4. Conclusions

As reviewed above, most of the recent studies on sound localization and lateralization have shown that performance with bilaterally fitted devices was better than that with unilaterally fitted device for bilateral (simulated) CHL. However, the judgment accuracy was generally lower than that for normal hearing, and the localization errors tended to be larger than for normal hearing. It should also be noted that the degree of accuracy in sound localization with bilateral BCDs varied considerably among patients. Many factors such as the type of device, the experimental conditions, participants, and pathways from the stimulus sound to both cochleae can affect the results. Especially, it is unclear whether localization with bilaterally fitted devices, for which the presentation level exceeds the threshold in bilateral (simulated) conductive hearing loss, involves both air-conducted sound and bone-conducted sound. Further research on sound localization is necessary to analyze the complicated mechanism of BC, including suprathreshold air conduction with bilateral devices.

Funding: This research received no external funding.

Institutional Review Board Statement: Not applicable.

Informed Consent Statement: Not applicable.

Data Availability Statement: Not applicable.

Acknowledgments: The author wishes to thank Gerard Remijn for helpful comments and English corrections on this review.

Conflicts of Interest: The author declares no conflict of interest.

Abbreviations

aBCD	adhesive bone conduction device
BAHA	bone-anchored hearing aid
BB	Bonebridge
BC	bone conduction
BCDs	bone conduction devices
BCHAs	bone conduction hearing aids
CCHAs	cartilage conduction hearing aids
CHL	conductive hearing loss
DM	directional microphone
HL	hearing level
HRTF	head-related transfer function
ILD	interaural level difference
ITD	interaural time difference
MAA	minimum audible angle
MAE	mean absolute localization error
μs	microsecond
RMSE	root mean square error
TA	transcranial attenuation
TD	transcranial delay

References

1. Moore, B.C.J. 7. Space perception. In *An Introduction to the Psychology of Hearing*, 5th ed.; Academic Press: San Diego, CA, USA, 2003; pp. 233–298.
2. Plack, C.J. 9. Spatial hearing. In *The Sense of Hearing*; Psychology Press: New York, NY, USA, 2005; pp. 173–192.
3. Bosman, A.J.; Snik, A.F.; van der Pouw, C.T.; Mylanus, E.A.; Cremers, C.W. Audiometric evaluation of bilaterally fitted bone-anchored hearing aids. *Audiology* **2001**, *40*, 158–167. [CrossRef]
4. Häusler, R.; Colburn, S.; Marr, E. Sound localization in subjects with impaired hearing. Spatial-discrimination and interaural-discrimination tests. *Acta Otolaryngol. Suppl.* **1983**, *400*, 1–62. [CrossRef]
5. Kramer, S.E.; Kapteyn, T.S.; Festen, J.M.; Tobi, H. Factors in subjective hearing disability. *Audiology* **1995**, *34*, 311–320. [CrossRef]
6. Kramer, S.E.; Kapteyn, T.S.; Festen, J.M. The self-reported handicapping effect of hearing disabilities. *Audiology* **1998**, *37*, 302–312. [CrossRef]
7. Littler, T.S.; Knight, J.J.; Strange, P.H. Hearing by bone conduction and the use of bone-conduction hearing aids. *Proc. R. Soc. Med.* **1952**, *45*, 783–790. [CrossRef]
8. Snik, A.F.M.; Beynon, A.J.; van der Pouw, C.T.M.; Mylanus, E.A.M.; Cremers, C.W.R.J. Binaural application of the bone-anchored hearing aid. *Ann Otol. Rhinol. Laryngol.* **1998**, *107*, 187–193. [CrossRef] [PubMed]
9. Tjellström, A.; Håkansson, B.; Lindström, J.; Brånemark, P.I.; Hallén, O.; Rosenhall, U.; Leijon, A. Analysis of the mechanical impedance of bone-anchored hearing aids. *Acta Otolaryngol.* **1980**, *89*, 85–92. [CrossRef] [PubMed]
10. Tjellström, A.; Granström, G. Long-term follow-up with the bone-anchored hearing aid: A review of the first 100 patients between 1977 and 1985. *Ear Nose Throat J.* **1994**, *73*, 112–114. [CrossRef] [PubMed]
11. Priwin, C.; Stenfelt, S.; Granström, G.; Tjellström, A.; Håkansson, B. Bilateral bone-anchored hearing aids (BAHAs): An audiometric evaluation. *Laryngoscope* **2004**, *114*, 77–84. [CrossRef] [PubMed]
12. Janssen, R.M.; Hong, P.; Chadha, N.K. Bilateral bone-anchored hearing aids for bilateral permanent conductive hearing loss: A systematic review. *Otolaryngol. Head Neck Surg.* **2012**, *147*, 412–422. [CrossRef] [PubMed]
13. Priwin, C.; Jönsson, R.; Hultcrantz, M.; Granström, G. BAHA in children and adolescents with unilateral or bilateral conductive hearing loss: A study of outcome. *Int. J. Pediatr. Otorhinolaryngol.* **2007**, *71*, 135–145. [CrossRef]
14. Kaga, K.; Setou, M.; Nakamura, M. Bone-conducted sound lateralization of interaural time difference and interaural intensity difference in children and a young adult with bilateral microtia and atresia of the ears. *Acta Otolaryngol.* **2001**, *121*, 274–277.
15. Schmerber, S.; Sheykholeslami, K.; Kermany, M.H.; Hotta, S.; Kaga, K. Time-intensity trading in bilateral congenital aural atresia patients. *Hear. Res.* **2005**, *202*, 248–257. [CrossRef]
16. Reinfeldt, S.; Håkansson, B.; Taghavi, H.; Olofsson, M.E. New developments in bone-conduction hearing implants: A review. *Med. Devices* **2015**, *8*, 79–93. [CrossRef] [PubMed]
17. ADHEAR. Available online: https://blog.medel.pro/adhear-hearing-system/ (accessed on 31 March 2021).
18. Hosoi, H.; Yanai, S.; Nishimura, T.; Sakaguchi, T.; Iwakura, T.; Yoshino, K. Development of cartilage conduction hearing aid. *Arch. Mater. Sci. Eng.* **2010**, *42*, 104–110.
19. Zeitooni, M.; Mäki-Torkko, E.; Stenfelt, S. Binaural hearing ability with bilateral bone conduction stimulation in subjects with normal hearing: Implications for bone conduction hearing aids. *Ear Hear.* **2016**, *37*, 690–702. [CrossRef] [PubMed]
20. Gatehouse, S.; Noble, W. The speech, spatial and qualities of hearing scale (SSQ). *Int J. Audiol.* **2004**, *43*, 85–99. [CrossRef] [PubMed]
21. Gawliczek, T.; Munzinger, F.; Anschuetz, L.; Caversaccio, M.; Kompis, M.; Wimmer, W. Unilateral and bilateral audiological benefit with an adhesively attached, noninvasive bone conduction hearing system. *Otol. Neurotol.* **2018**, *39*, 1025–1030. [CrossRef]
22. Gawliczek, T.; Wimmer, W.; Munzinger, F.; Caversaccio, M.; Kompis, M. Speech understanding and sound localization with a new nonimplantable wearing option for Baha. *BioMed. Res. Int.* **2018**, *2018*, 5264124. [CrossRef]
23. Snapp, H.; Vogt, K.; Agterberg, M.J.H. Bilateral bone conduction stimulation provides reliable binaural cues for localization. *Hear. Res.* **2020**, *388*, 107881. [CrossRef]
24. Dun, C.A.J.; Agterberg, M.J.; Cremers, C.W.; Hol, M.K.; Snik, A.F. Bilateral bone conduction devices: Improved hearing ability in children with bilateral conductive hearing loss. *Ear Hear.* **2013**, *34*, 806–808. [CrossRef] [PubMed]
25. Fan, X.; Ping, L.; Yang, T.; Niu, X.; Chen, Y.; Xia, X.; Gao, R.; Fan, Y.; Chen, X. Comparative effects of unilateral and bilateral bone conduction hearing devices on functional hearing and sound localization abilities in patients with bilateral microtia-atresia. *Acta Otolaryngol.* **2020**, *140*, 575–582. [CrossRef]
26. Besten, C.A.D.; Vogt, K.; Bosman, A.J.; Snik, A.F.M.; Hol, M.K.S.; Agterberg, M.J.H. The merits of bilateral application of bone-conduction devices in children with bilateral conductive hearing loss. *Ear Hear.* **2020**, *41*, 1327–1332. [CrossRef] [PubMed]
27. Nishimura, T.; Hosoi, H.; Saito, O.; Shimokura, R.; Yamanaka, T.; Kitahara, T. Sound localisation ability using cartilage conduction hearing aids in bilateral aural atresia. *Int. J. Audiol.* **2020**, *59*, 891–896. [CrossRef]
28. Ren, L.; Duan, Z.; Yu, J.; Xie, Y.; Zhang, T. Instant auditory benefit of an adhesive BCHD on children with bilateral congenital microtia. *Clin. Otolaryngol.* **2021**, *46*, 1089–1094. [CrossRef] [PubMed]
29. Caspers, C.J.I.; Janssen, A.M.; Agterberg, M.J.H.; Cremers, C.W.R.J.; Hol, M.K.S.; Bosman, A.J. Sound localization with bilateral bone conduction devices. *Eur. Arch. Otorhinolaryngol.* **2021**. [CrossRef]

30. Sakai, Y.; Karino, S.; Kaga, K. Bone-conducted auditory brainstem-evoked responses and skull vibratory velocity measurement in rats at frequencies of 0.5–30 kHz with a new giant magnetostrictive bone conduction transducer. *Acta Otolaryngol.* **2016**, *126*, 926–933. [CrossRef]
31. Zahorik, P.; Bangayan, P.; Sundareswaran, V.; Wang, K.; Tam, C. Perceptual recalibration in human sound localization: Learning to remediate front-back reversals. *J. Acoust Soc. Am.* **2006**, *120*, 343–359. [CrossRef]
32. ADHEAR SYSTEM Including the ADHEAR Audio Processor and the ADHEAR Adhesive Adapter Technical Data. Available online: https://s3.medel.com/pdf/28867_40_ADHEAR_Factsheet_English.pdf (accessed on 31 March 2021).
33. Cochlear™ Baha®5 Sound Processor Data Sheet. Available online: https://www.cochlear.com/3116aa05-0d7d-4806-9ed4-7ddb058d8998/BUN335-ISS2-OCT17-Baha5-SP-Datasheet.pdf?MOD=AJPERES&CVID=nlcuPdQ (accessed on 31 March 2021).
34. Cire, G. The Baha 5 Sound Processor Overview. *Audio Online*, 2015. Available online: https://www.audiologyonline.com/articles/baha-5-sound-processor-overview-14427 (accessed on 23 July 2021).
35. The Bonebridge™ Bone Conduction Implant System Data Sheet. Available online: https://s3.medel.com/pdf/INT/professionals_brochure2014.pdf (accessed on 31 March 2021).
36. Shimokura, R.; Hosoi, H.; Iwakura, T.; Nishimura, T.; Matsui, T. Development of monaural and binaural behind-the-ear cartilage conduction hearing aids. *Appl. Acoust* **2013**, *74*, 1234–1240. [CrossRef]
37. Denk, F.; Ewert, S.D.; Kollmeier, B. On the limitations of sound localization with hearing devices. *J. Acoust Soc. Am.* **2019**, *146*, 1732–1744. [CrossRef]
38. Keidser, G.; Rohrseitz, K.; Dillon, H.; Hamacher, V.; Carter, L.; Rass, U.; Convery, E. The effect of multi-channel wide dynamic range compression, noise reduction, and the dsirectional microphone on horizontal localization performance in hearing aid wearers. *Int. J. Audiol.* **2006**, *45*, 563–579. [CrossRef]
39. Van den Bogaert, T.; Klasen, T.J.; Moonen, M.; Van Deun, L.; Wouters, J. Horizontal localization with bilateral hearing aids: Without is better than with. *J. Acoust Soc. Am.* **2006**, *119*, 515–526. [CrossRef]
40. Ibrahim, I.; Parsa, V.; Macpherson, E.; Cheesman, M. Evaluation of speech intelligibility and sound localization abilities with hearing aids using binaural wireless technology. *Audiol. Res.* **2013**, *3*, e1. [CrossRef] [PubMed]
41. Johnson, J.A.; Xu, J.; Cox, R.M. Impact of Hearing Aid Technology on Outcomes in Daily Life III: Localization. *Ear Hear.* **2017**, *38*, 746–759. [CrossRef]
42. Stenfelt, S. Transcranial attenuation of bone-conducted sound when stimulation is at the mastoid and at the bone conduction hearing aid position. *Otol. Neurotol.* **2012**, *33*, 105–114. [CrossRef]
43. Dobrev, I.; Stenfelt, S.; Röösli, C.; Bolt, L.; Pfiffner, F.; Gerig, R.; Huber, A.; Sim, J.H. Influence of stimulation position on the sensitivity for bone conduction hearing aids without skin penetration. *Int. J. Audiol.* **2016**, *55*, 439–446. [CrossRef]
44. Asakura, T.; Takai, K. Effect of the contact condition of the actuator on the sound localization of bone-conducted reproduction. *Acoust Sci. Technol* **2019**, *40*, 259–264. [CrossRef]
45. Middlebrooks, J.C.; Green, D.M. Sound localization by human listeners. *Annu Rev. Psychol.* **1991**, *42*, 135–159. [CrossRef] [PubMed]
46. Butler, R.A. The bandwidth effect on monaural and binaural localization. *Hear. Res.* **1986**, *21*, 67–73. [CrossRef]
47. Mills, A.W. On the minimum audible angle. *J. Acoust Soc. Am.* **1958**, *30*, 237–246. [CrossRef]
48. Lovett, R.E.S.; Kitterick, P.T.; Huang, S.; Summerfield, A.Q. The developmental trajectory of spatial listening skills in normal-hearing children. *J. Speech Lang. Hear. Res.* **2012**, *55*, 865–878. [CrossRef]
49. Asp, F.; Olofsson, Å.; Berninger, E. Corneal-reflection eye-tracking technique for the assessment of horizontal sound localization accuracy from 6 months of age. *Ear Hear.* **2016**, *37*, e104–e118. [CrossRef]
50. Yost, W.A.; Zhong, X. Sound source localization identification accuracy: Bandwidth dependencies. *J. Acoust Soc. Am.* **2014**, *136*, 2737–2746. [CrossRef]
51. Rakerd, B.; Hartmann, W.M. Localization of sound in rooms, III: Onset and duration effects. *J. Acoust Soc. Am.* **1986**, *80*, 1695–1706. [CrossRef]
52. Asp, F.; Jakobsson, A.; Berminger, E. The effect of simulated unilateral hearing loss on horizontal sound localization accuracy and recognition of speech in spatially separate competing speech. *Hear. Res.* **2018**, *357*, 54–63. [CrossRef] [PubMed]
53. Kaga, K.; Asato, H. Sound lateralization test in patients with unilateral microtia and atresia after reconstruction of the auricle and external canal and fitting of canal-type hearing aids. *Acta Otolaryngol.* **2016**, *136*, 368–372. [CrossRef] [PubMed]
54. Studebaker, G.A. Clinical masking of the nontest ear. *J. Speech Hear. Disord* **1967**, *32*, 360–371. [CrossRef]
55. Kaga, M. Development of sound localization. *Acta Paediatr. Jpn.* **1992**, *34*, 134–138. [CrossRef]
56. Firszt, J.B.; Reeder, R.M.; Dwyer, N.Y.; Burton, H.; Holden, L.K. Localization training results in individuals with unilateral severe to profound hearing loss. *Hear. Res.* **2015**, *319*, 48–55. [CrossRef]
57. Klumpp, R.G.; Eady, H.R. Some measurements of interaural time difference thresholds. *J. Acoust Soc. Am.* **1956**, *28*, 859–860. [CrossRef]
58. Eeg-Olofsson, M. Transmission of Bone-Conducted Sound in the Human Skull Based on Vibration and Perceptual Measures. 2012. Available online: https://gupea.ub.gu.se/bitstream/2077/28248/1/gupea_2077_28248_1.pdf (accessed on 31 March 2021).
59. Stenfelt, S.; Zeitooni, M. Binaural hearing ability with mastoid applied bilateral bone conduction stimulation in normal hearing subjects. *J. Acoust Soc. Am.* **2013**, *134*, 481–493. [CrossRef] [PubMed]
60. Röösli, C.; Dobrev, I.; Pfiffner, F. Transcranial attenuation in bone conduction stimulation. *Ear Hear.* **2021**, in press.

61. Franke, E.K. Response of the human skull to mechanical vibrations. *J. Acoust Soc. Am.* **1956**, *28*, 1277–1284. [CrossRef]
62. Wigand, M.E.; Borucki, H.J.; Schmitt, H.G. Bone Conduction of sound pulse waves. Physical measurement of velocity. *Acta Otolaryngol.* **1964**, *58*, 95–104. (In German) [CrossRef] [PubMed]
63. Tonndorf, J.; Jahn, A.F. Velocity of propagation of bone-conducted sound in a human head. *J. Acoust Soc. Am.* **1981**, *70*, 1294–1297. [CrossRef]
64. Stenfelt, S.; Goode, R.L. Transmission properties of bone conducted sound: Measurements in cadaver heads. *J. Acoust Soc. Am.* **2005**, *118*, 2373–2391. [CrossRef]
65. Farrell, N.F.; Hartl, R.M.B.; Benichoux, V.; Brown, A.D.; Cass, S.P.; Tollin, D.J. Intracochlear measurements of interaural time and level differences conveyed by bilateral bone conduction systems. *Otol. Neurotol.* **2017**, *38*, 1476–1483. [CrossRef] [PubMed]

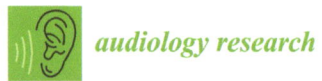 audiology research

Review

Perception Mechanism of Bone-Conducted Ultrasound and Its Clinical Use

Tadashi Nishimura [1,*], Tadao Okayasu [1], Akinori Yamashita [1], Hiroshi Hosoi [2] and Tadashi Kitahara [1]

[1] Department of Otolaryngology-Head and Neck Surgery, Nara Medical University, 840 Shijo-cho, Kashihara, Nara 634-8522, Japan; tokayasu@naramed-u.ac.jp (T.O.); akinori@naramed-u.ac.jp (A.Y.); tkitahara@naramed-u.ac.jp (T.K.)

[2] MBT (Medicine-Based Town) Institute, Nara Medical University, 840 Shijo-cho, Kashihara, Nara 634-8522, Japan; hosoi@naramed-u.ac.jp

* Correspondence: t-nishim@naramed-u.ac.jp; Tel.: +81-744-22-3051

Abstract: It is generally believed that ultrasound cannot be heard. However, ultrasound is audible when it is presented through bone conduction. Bone-conducted ultrasound (BCU) has unique characteristics; the most interesting is its perception in patients with profound deafness. Some patients can perceive it and discriminate speech-modulated BCU. Previous reports have suggested that BCU can be used for a hearing aid or tinnitus sound therapy. In this review, the perception of BCU at both the peripheral and central levels was investigated based on previous studies, although some of them remain controversial. We also investigated the clinical use of BCU. To develop hearing aids utilizing BCU, the encoding of speech signals into BCU has to be established. The outcomes of the reported speech modulations were evaluated. Furthermore, the suppression of tinnitus by BCU was reviewed, and the feasibility of the application of BCU to tinnitus treatment was investigated.

Keywords: bone conduction; ultrasound; ultrasonic perception; high frequency sound; profound deaf; tinnitus

1. Introduction

The audible frequency range of the human ear is between 16 Hz and 24 kHz [1], and a sound above this frequency range is referred to as "ultrasound." In contrast, ultrasound, whose frequency ranges up to at least 120 kHz, can create an auditory sensation when delivered via bone conduction (BC) [2–4]. Previous studies indicated that middle ear impedance might prevent ultrasound transmission via air conduction (AC) [3,5]. Other previous studies have suggested the generation of audible sound due to a nonlinear process in BC [4,6]. If a generated audible sound is predominantly associated with the perception of bone-conducted ultrasound (BCU), the characteristics of the induced sensation should resemble those of the audible sound. However, the reported characteristics of BCU perception (ultrasonic perception) are unique and not always observed with the perception of air-conducted audible sound (ACAS). In this review, ACAS was defined as an audible sound to avoid confusion in terminology. "Audible sound" was used for ACAS and distinguished from "ultrasound," although ultrasound is audible via BC.

2. Characteristics of Ultrasonic Perception

According to previous reports, the pitch of BCU resembles that of ACAS at frequencies of 8–16 kHz, independent of its own frequencies [3,4,6]. The dynamic range is very narrow and similar to that obtained in patients with a cochlear implant [7]. The most interesting unique characteristic is the perception in patients with profound deafness. Some of them can perceive BCU [8–10], which suggests the contribution of a unique perception mechanism different from that of ACAS. Lenhart et al. found that some patients with severe hearing loss could discriminate BCU stimuli modulated with speech [8]. Cochlear implants are usually required in patients with profound deafness [11,12]. If a speech signal is delivered with an ultrasonic hearing device, a profoundly deaf individual can recover speech perception without any surgical operation. To apply this method in clinical practice, the mechanism underlying its perception should be established.

3. Peripheral Perception Mechanism of BCU

For audible sound, the presentation of an acoustic stimulus can disturb the perception of other sounds (masking), and the amount of masking grows as the difference between the frequencies of the two sounds reduces. The masking of ACAS by BCU can be used to establish its perception mechanism. In our previous study, ACAS at frequencies below 8 kHz was not masked by BCU, which suggested that ultrasonic perception was not significantly associated with the perception of ACAS at frequencies of ≤ 8 kHz [7]. In contrast, the threshold of high-frequency ACAS (above 8 kHz) was remarkably elevated under a low-sensation level (SL) BCU presentation. With a 5-dB SL BCU presentation, the maximum amount of the masking was recognized at approximately 30 dB at 14 kHz. The peak of the masking patterns occurred between 10 and 14 kHz, which was independent of the ultrasound frequency [7]. Furthermore, the increase in BCU masker to 10 dB SL induced greater masking. Masking increases faster than linearly, showing a rate of 2–5.8 dB/dB between 9 and 15 kHz, and the maximum growth was observed at 10 kHz. For ACAS, an increase in masking of more than 1 dB/1 dB can be observed when the masker frequency is lower than that of the signal [13]. If the current masking were produced by a demodulated sound, the characteristic frequency of the modulated sound would be below 10 kHz. However, it was lower than the peak of masking patterns. Thus, it appears that the observed masking was not produced by the demodulated sound but by the ultrasound itself. Nakagawa et al. measured the vibration of the eardrum with a laser Doppler when ultrasound was presented using BC [14]. No significant generation of the demodulated audible sound was identified, and they concluded that nonlinear distortion does not contribute to perception. Considering the responsivity of the outer hair cells (OHCs) to the ultrasonic frequency range, the active process derived from OHCs cannot probably function during ultrasonic perception. According to Bekesy's traveling wave theory [15], ultrasound causes the largest vibration amplitude at locations basal to those responding maximally to high-frequency ACAS. If the theory were applied to the vibrations of the basilar membrane produced by BCU, they would become stronger and spread downward as intensity increases, which probably produces both masking of high-frequency ACAS and generation of auditory sensation [7].

If the peripheral perception organ of BCU is located in the cochlea, ultrasonic perception may be possible to be completely masked by ACAS. In previous studies, ultrasonic perception was barely masked by ACAS [4,16]. However, given the masking produced by BCU, ultrasonic perception is most likely associated with high-frequency ACAS perception [7]. If the masking spectrum does not sufficiently cover its frequency range, the ultrasonic perception cannot be masked. BCU can excite a broad cochlear region, considering the masking pattern of ACAS produced by BCU [7]. When the intensity of the ACAS masker is sufficiently high, the excitation spreads broadly depending on the intensity. An ACAS that excites a sufficient cochlear region can mask the ultrasonic perception. Our previous study found that ultrasonic perception was masked by high-frequency ACAS, especially when the masker frequency and intensity were 10–14 kHz and above 80 dB SPL, respectively [17]. The frequency of an ACAS masker, which could mask ultrasonic perception, was equal to that of an ACAS, which was strongly masked by BCU [7]. Consequently, it is suggested that ultrasonic perception is associated with a high-frequency ACAS perception, and both perceptions may have common auditory pathways. Figure 1 shows a schematic of the mechanism of ultrasonic perception and masking. Our studies on masking produced by BCU and masking of ultrasonic perception by ACAS corroborated our hypothesis.

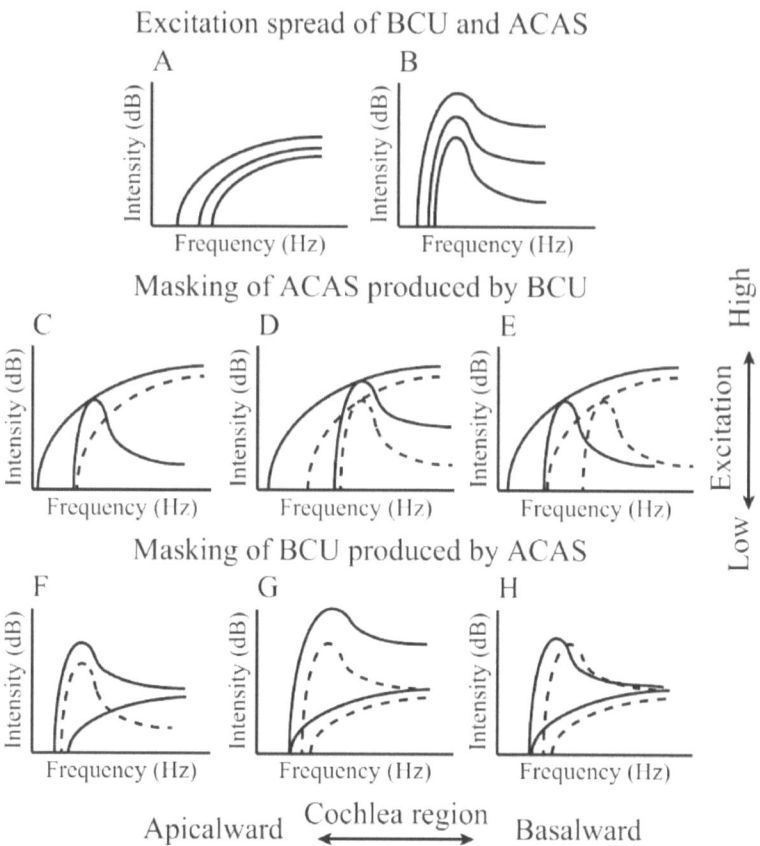

Figure 1. Schema of the excitation pattern and growth of masking by bone-conducted ultrasound (BCU) and air-conducted audible sound (ACAS). Parts (**A**,**B**) indicate the excitation pattern depending on the intensity. For BCU, the excitation does not show a sharp peak and spreads fast to the apical ward (Part (**A**)). For ACAS, the excitation pattern shows a peak at the characteristic frequency and spreads slowly to the apical ward (Part (**B**)). Part (**C**) indicates masking of ACAS by BCU. ACAS cannot be masked with a low-level masker (dashed line). However, when the excitation by BCU covers that by ACAS (solid line), ACAS is masked. Parts (**D**,**E**) indicate the growth of masking depending on the intensity. The dashed and solid lines indicate the masking pattern observed at a low- or high-level masker, respectively. The masking grows fast (Part (**D**)) and also spreads fast to the apical ward (Part (**E**)). In contrast, Part (**F**) indicates masking of BCU by ACAS. At low ACAS masker intensity (dashed line), the excitation pattern shows a sharp peak. Because BCU excites a broad cochlear region, ACAS below 60 dB SPL cannot mask BCU. When the masker intensity is sufficiently large (solid line), the excitation by ACAS covers a broad cochlear region and masks BCU. Parts (**G**,**H**) indicate the growth of masking, depending on the intensity. The dashed and solid lines indicate the masking at low and high signal intensities, respectively. The excitation by BCU fast spreads to the apical ward. Accordingly, a large increase in masker intensity (Part (**G**)) or masker frequency shift to the lower frequency range (Part (**H**)) is required for masking. In each schema, vertical and horizontal axes indicate the excitation and cochlear region, respectively. (Figure 1 was originally presented in Nishimura et al. 2011, Figure 1 [17]).

In our hypothesis of the peripheral perception mechanism, the function of OHCs does not contribute to ultrasonic perception. Inner hair cell (IHC) activity induced by ultrasound plays an important role in ultrasonic perception, even without the presence of modulation, and it does not depend on the enhancement of BCU by OHCs in the basal turn of the cochlea. Regarding the thresholds of BCU in patients with hearing impairment, no patients with an estimated total loss of the IHC system in the cochlear basal turn could hear BCU [17]. A significant relationship was found between BCU thresholds and the estimated extent of the presence of IHC function in the cochlea. In another study, the impact of cisplatin administration on the thresholds of ACAS and BCU was evaluated in patients with head and neck cancer [18]. Ototoxic drugs, such as cisplatin usually induce hearing deficits predominantly due to the disorder of OHCs [19]. The damage to OHCs can induce the threshold elevations of ACAS, and the thresholds of BCU can be maintained owing to the independence of the OHC function. In the results, although the thresholds for high-frequency ACAS significantly worsened after treatment, the thresholds of BCU did not increase [18]. These findings are consistent with our hypothesis for the perception mechanisms. With the findings in the previous studies, the peripheral perception mechanism has been gradually revealed but remains controversial.

4. Ultrasonic Perception at the Central Level

In previous studies on ultrasonic perception at the central level, neural activation was observed with magnetoencephalography and positron emission tomography in the auditory cortex but not in the somatosensory cortex [9,10]. These findings objectively established that ultrasonic perception is an auditory sensation, not a somatosensory sensation. Previous studies evaluated N1m responses evoked by BCU and compared them with those for ACAS [20–25]. These studies demonstrated several differences between the characteristics of ACAS and BCU, suggesting a unique mechanism underlying the perception of BCU at the central level. The magnitude of N1m grows as a function of intensity and duration [21,24]. The growth rates of N1m amplitude are differed for ACAS and BCU, which may be associated with a narrow dynamic range of ultrasonic perception. However, the growth of the N1m amplitude was saturated approximately at the uncomfortable loudness level or the duration of 40 ms for both stimuli [22,24]. Regarding the detection of the frequency difference, the mismatch field (MMF) evoked by the frequency change for BCU was significantly lower than that for ACAS [23]. Considering the peripheral mechanism, excited cochlear regions depend on intensity but not frequency [17]. Therefore, distinguishing the frequency of BCU is difficult. The unique characteristics of the central auditory response for BCU may be explained by the differences in the peripheral perception mechanism. The fundamental neural system at the central level is probably similar to that of ACAS. Further studies are required for the establishment of ultrasonic perception at the central level as well as the peripheral.

5. Clinical Use of Ultrasonic Perception

One of the clinical applications of ultrasonic perception is hearing aids for profound deafness. Some characteristics of ultrasonic perception resemble those of the perception provided with a cochlear implant rather than those of ACAS perception. The most pertinent difference between BCU and cochlear implants is the spectral resolution. BCU can stimulate one broad cochlear region in the basal turn, which can be considered a single-channel hearing device, whereas cochlear implants have multiple channels [26–28]. Speech has to be encoded by ultrasound for communication using this single channel. The role of the temporal fine structure and envelope is important for the perception of speech [29,30]. Previous studies employed amplification modulation as the encoding method [31–33]. During the encoding process, speech is used as a carrier sound, and BCU is modulated with this carrier. The envelope of the speech-modulated BCU can transmit cues for speech recognition.

6. Recognition of Speech-Modulated BCU in Normal-Hearing Individuals

In previous studies, speech-modulated BCU facilitated good speech recognition scores for participants with normal hearing [31–33]. These results are interesting because the speech-modulated BCU was accurately recognized without any training. Demodulation in the nonlinear process is probably associated with high recognition scores [34]. Fujimoto et al. evaluated the difference limens for frequency of BCU modulated by air-conducted pure tones under two conditions: using amplitude modulation based on a double-side-band transmitted carrier and a suppressed carrier [35]. Comparing the pitches of these conditions, they demonstrated a nonlinear process underlying the perception of modulated BCU.

Changes in voice pitch contribute to communication. During conversation, speech sounds convey both linguistic and non-linguistic information, such as attitudes and emotions. Prosody is important for the conveyance of information, such as questions or affirmations, through speech and the expression of emotions. In a previous behavioral study, prosodic information for speech-modulated BCU could also be distinguished during normal hearing [36]. Furthermore, prosodic discrimination for speech-modulated BCU was objectively evaluated by measuring the MMFs elicited by prosodic and segmental changes [37]. In almost all the participants, prominent MMF was elicited by prosodic and segmental changes in speech-modulated BCU. Although the discrimination of speech-modulated BCU is slightly inferior to that of air-conducted speech, prosodic change can be distinguished to the same degree as segmental change, even for speech-modulated BCU.

7. Recognition of Speech-Modulated BCU in Hearing-Impaired Patients

If demodulation works in the perception of speech modulated BCU, good speech recognition without any training by participants with normal hearing can be explained without difficulty. BCU modulated by speech signals may be demodulated into original signals, and, consequently, most participants would be able to recognize them. In contrast, this also means that hearing-impaired patients, especially profoundly deaf patients, cannot recognize any speech signals because demodulated audible sound cannot be recognized because of their hearing disorder. In contrast, Lenhart et al. reported the discrimination of speech-modulated BCU in patients with severe hearing loss [8]. Hosoi objectively demonstrated the perception of speech-modulated BCU in hearing-impaired patients using MEG [9]. Regarding N1m evoked by speech-modulated BCU in individuals with normal hearing, the impact of the duration of speech-modulated BCU on the N1m amplitude and latency was different from that of AC speech [38]. These results suggest that N1m evoked by speech-modulated BCU is influenced mainly by the ultrasonic component as well as the demodulated audible sound. Both the signal and carrier are associated with the perception, and the discrimination cue of the original speech signal is obtained from the demodulated signal in individuals with normal hearing. By suppressing the perception of demodulated sounds, the responses to the BCU components may be evaluated. Since BCU is difficult to mask by ACAS with a frequency of ≤ 8 kHz [7], demodulated sound can be masked by an ACAS masker with the minimum effect of ultrasonic perception. The results obtained can be utilized for the development of hearing devices in patients with hearing impairment.

Our previous study investigated the intelligibility of speech-modulated BCU using a numeral word list under masking conditions [39]. In the presence of masking, the speech recognition curve for the original speech signal shifted to the right, depending on the masker intensity. In contrast, while masking influences the intelligibility of the speech-modulated BCU, the curve did not shift upward, which was similar to the original speech signal (Figure 2). These differences in the masking effect suggest that the recognition of speech-modulated BCU differs from that of the original speech signal. If recognition is performed solely by demodulation, the recognition curve shifts upward depending on the masking intensity. The difference between the results for speech-modulated BCU and the original speech signal indicated the importance of direct ultrasonic stimulation, particularly under the masking condition. The characteristics of the confusion pattern for speech-modulated BCU were different from those of the original speech signal depending on the masker intensity. The frequency of confusion of some words correlated positively with increasing masker intensity (Figure 3). Under high-intensity masking conditions, the demodulated sound is strongly masked by the speech-weighted noise; therefore, participants are forced to respond based on the unmasked ultrasonic stimulation. The previous findings indicated the difference between speech-modulated BCU and the original speech signal and showed that direct ultrasonic stimulation, as well as demodulated sound, contributed to recognition. However, the current data also suggest that information transmitted solely by ultrasonic stimulation is insufficient to recognize the conversation. A good speech recognition score is probably difficult to obtain with the present BCU device in profoundly deaf patients. To improve the benefits, visual information may facilitate communication with an ultrasonic hearing device [33]. Additional developments are necessary for clinical applications.

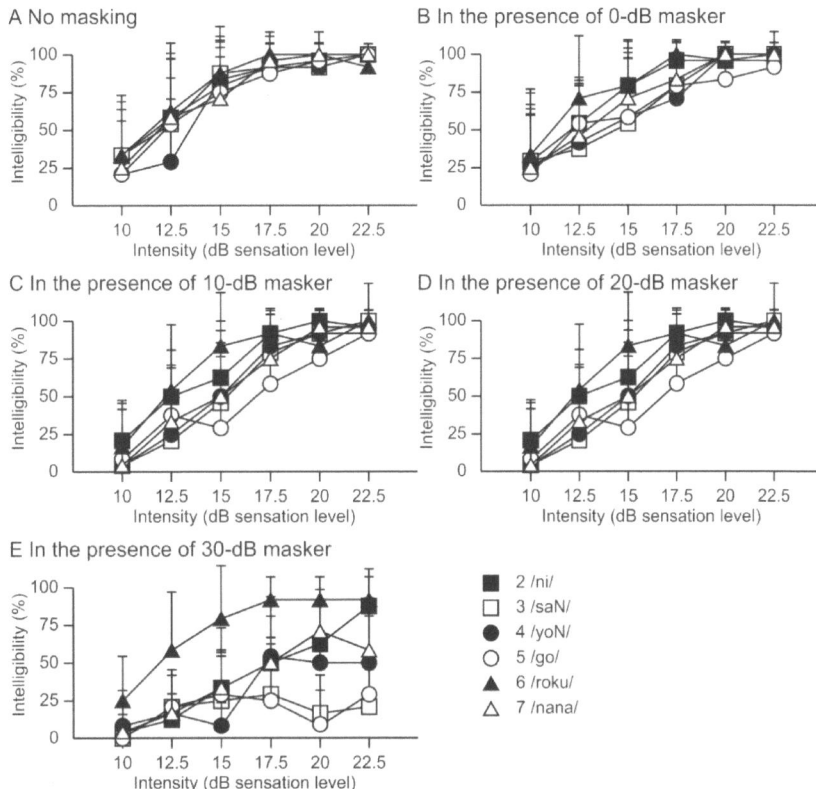

Figure 2. The average scores for the correct answers for each masker condition. The intelligibility of speech-modulated 30 kHz BCU was measured under five masking conditions in eight normal hearing volunteers. A numeral word list was used as speech materials. The ultrasonic transducer was fixed on the forehead. A speech-weighted noise was employed as masking and binaurally presented using earphones. The scores decreased as the masker intensity increased. The reduction in the scores showed variations among the stimuli. The vertical bars indicate standard deviations. (Figure 2 was originally presented in Nishimura et al. 2014, Figure 6 [39]).

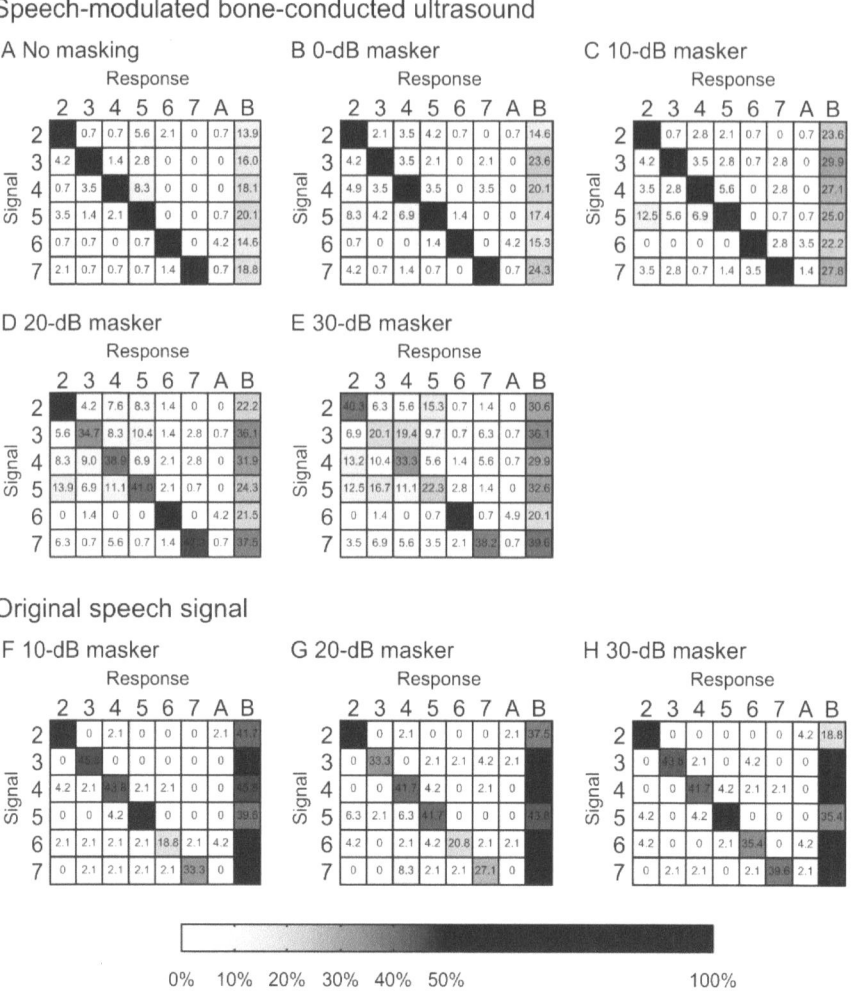

Figure 3. Confusion matrices based on the results of speech-modulated bone-conducted ultrasound (**A–E**) and original speech signals (**F–H**) under different masking conditions. The results were obtained in the above-mentioned eight normal hearing volunteers. Presentation signals are represented on the left axis and responses across the top axis. "A" and "B" indicate other responses besides the six numeral words and no response, respectively. Blocks with larger grey values (i.e., darker shading) indicate higher appearance frequencies for those pairs. When the appearance frequency was higher than 50%, the block is marked fully black. Numerical values in the cells indicate the percentage of the appearance frequency. (Figure 3 was originally presented in Nishimura et al. 2014, Figure 10 [39]).

8. Application of BCU for Tinnitus Treatment

Tinnitus is a common audiological disease, and the prevalence of continuous subjective tinnitus among adults ranges from 5.1% to 42.7% [40]. It negatively affects the quality of life [41], and the prevalence of depressive disorders in this population can be high, ranging from 10% to 90% [42]. However, the efficacy of pharmacological and behavioral interventions remains limited. Sound therapy and psychological approaches have become mainstream for treatment [43,44]. In sound therapy, patients regularly hear sounds using sound applications or sound devices, such as hearing aids, sound masking generators, or modified-sound/Notched-music devices [45]. These sound therapies cannot be conducted in patients with profound deafness due to the severity of their hearing deficits. In contrast, BCU may be utilized for sound therapy in patients with profound deafness because some of them can hear BCU [8–10]. In contrast with hearing aids, the predominant aim of sound therapy is the mitigation of the symptoms, not the improvement of speech recognition. Thus, BCU is available more easily for sound therapy in patients with severe hearing loss.

Tinnitus is temporarily masked by presenting a sound, and it is continuously reduced or disappears during the few seconds or minutes after the offset of the masker presentation. This continuous reduction or disappearance of tinnitus is referred to as residual inhibition (RI). RI has been regarded as a clinical index that reflects the degree of tinnitus inhibition [46]. Goldstein et al. found that 20–26 kHz BCU masked tinnitus in 52 patients [47]. They suggested that BCU may be effective in masking tinnitus [48]. However, they did not measure the RI. Koizumi et al. evaluated the RI induced by BCU in 21 patients with tinnitus [49]. The masker intensities of the 30-kHz BCU and audible sounds were set at the minimum masking levels of tinnitus plus 3 dB and 10 dB, respectively. The duration of RI induced by the 30-kHz BCU was significantly longer than that of the RI induced by the 4-kHz sounds. The peripheral stimulation characteristic of BCU probably contributed to inducing long RI durations. Considering the lower presentation of the BCU masker, these findings suggest that BCU suppresses tinnitus more effectively than ACAS.

Sound therapy is regularly administered during daily life. When a sound generation device is used for sound therapy, a generated sound is presented with an earphone for a defined therapy session. During the session, hearing can be disturbed by the generated sound. However, if BCU is used as the presented sound, it rarely affects hearing within the frequency range involved in daily conversation. In addition, ultrasound is delivered via BC, and the insertion of an earphone is not required. Thus, sound therapy utilizing BCU may minimize its influence on daily life and provide good benefits. Further studies on tinnitus therapy using BCU are required.

9. Conclusions

BCU is perceived in the basal turn of the cochlea. However, its perception mechanism is different from that of ACAS. The intelligibility for the speech-modulated BCU is comparable to that for the original speech signal in normal-hearing individuals due to the contribution of demodulation. Unfortunately, the lack of the contribution of demodulation to speech perception has to be taken into consideration in hearing impairment patients. The performance of the reported speech-modulated BCU in speech recognition is limited in patients with profound deafness, and further innovation may be required for clinical use. Regarding the application to tinnitus treatment, BCU devices have unique advantages. Unfortunately, the knowledge of BCU in this field has not been sufficient, and further study is required for its establishment.

Author Contributions: Drafting the manuscript: T.N., T.O., A.Y., Revising the manuscript: H.H., T.K., Approval of the manuscript: H.H., T.K. All authors have read and agreed to the published version of the manuscript.

Funding: Not applicable.

Institutional Review Board Statement: Not applicable.

Informed Consent Statement: Not applicable.

Data Availability Statement: Not applicable.

Conflicts of Interest: The authors declare no conflict of interest.

References

1. Wegel, R.P. Physical data and physiology of excitation of the auditory nerve. *Anns. Otol. Rhinol. Lar.* **1932**, *41*, 740–799. [CrossRef]
2. Gavreau, V. Audibillite de sons de frequence elevee. *Compt. Rendu.* **1948**, *226*, 2053–2054.
3. Pumphrey, R. Upper limit of frequency for human hearing. *Nature* **1950**, *166*, 571. [CrossRef] [PubMed]

4. Dieroff, H.G.; Ertel, H. Some thoughts on the perception of ultrasonics by man. *Arch. Otorhinolaryngol.* **1975**, *209*, 277–299. [CrossRef]
5. Corso, J.F. Bone-conduction thresholds for sonic and ultrasonic frequencies. *J. Acoust. Soc. Am.* **1963**, *35*, 1738–1743. [CrossRef]
6. Haeff, A.V.; Knox, C. Perception of ultrasound. *Science* **1963**, *139*, 590–592. [CrossRef]
7. Nishimura, T.; Nakagawa, S.; Sakaguchi, T.; Hosoi, H. Ultrasonic masker clarifies ultrasonic perception in man. *Hear. Res.* **2003**, *175*, 171–177. [CrossRef]
8. Lenhardt, M.L.; Skellett, R.; Wang, P.; Clarke, A.M. Human ultrasonic speech perception. *Science* **1991**, *253*, 82–85. [CrossRef]
9. Hosoi, H.; Imaizumi, S.; Sakaguchi, T.; Tonoike, M.; Murata, K. Activation of the auditory cortex by ultrasound. *Lancet* **1998**, *351*, 496–497. [CrossRef]
10. Imaizumi, S.; Hosoi, H.; Sakaguchi, T.; Watanabe, Y.; Sadato, N.; Nakamura, S.; Waki, A.; Yonekura, Y. Ultrasound activates the auditory cortex of profound deaf subjects. *NeuroReport* **2001**, *12*, 583–586. [CrossRef] [PubMed]
11. Carlson, M.L. Cochlear Implantation in Adults. *N. Engl. J. Med.* **2020**, *382*, 1531–1542. [CrossRef] [PubMed]
12. Lieu, J.E.C.; Kenna, M.; Anne, S.; Davidson, L. Hearing Loss in Children: A Review. *JAMA* **2020**, *324*, 2195–2205. [CrossRef] [PubMed]
13. Oxenham, A.J.; Micheyl, C.; Keebler, M.V.; Loper, A.; Santurette, S. Pitch perception beyond the traditional existence region of pitch. *Proc. Natl. Acad. Sci. USA* **2011**, *108*, 7629–7634. [CrossRef] [PubMed]
14. Nakagawa, S.; Ito, K. Mechanisms of Bone-conducted Ultrasonic Perception Assessed by Measurements of Acoustic Fields in the Outer Ear Canal and Vibrations of the Tympanic Membrane. *Annu. Int. Conf. IEEE Eng. Med. Biol. Soc.* **2018**, *2018*, 5962–5965. [CrossRef]
15. Von Békésy, G. *Experiments in Hearing*; McGraw-Hill: New York, NY, USA, 1960.
16. Bellucci, R.; Schuneider, D. Some observations on ultrasonic perception in man. *Ann. Otol. Rhinol. Laryngol.* **1962**, *71*, 719–726. [CrossRef]
17. Nishimura, T.; Okayasu, T.; Uratani, Y.; Fukuda, F.; Saito, O.; Hosoi, H. Peripheral perception mechanism of ultrasonic hearing. *Hear. Res.* **2011**, *277*, 176–183. [CrossRef]
18. Okayasu, T.; Nishimura, T.; Yamashita, A.; Saito, O.; Fukuda, F.; Yanai, S.; Hosoi, H. Human ultrasonic hearing is induced by a direct ultrasonic stimulation of the cochlea. *Neurosci. Lett.* **2013**, *539*, 71–76. [CrossRef] [PubMed]
19. Borse, V.A.; Aameri, R.F.H.; Sheehan, K.; Sheth, S.; Kaur, T.; Mukherjea, D.; Tupal, S.; Lowy, M.; Ghosh, S.; Dhukhwa, A.; et al. Epigallocatechin-3-gallate, a prototypic chemopreventative agent for protection against cisplatin-based ototoxicity. *Cell Death Dis.* **2017**, *8*, e2921. [CrossRef]
20. Sakaguchi, T.; Hirano, T.; Nishimura, T.; Nakagawa, S.; Watanabe, Y.; Hosoi, H.; Imaizumi, S.; Tonoike, M. Cerebral neuromagnetic responses evoked by two-channel bone-conducted ultrasound stimuli. In *Proceedings of the 12th International Conference on Biomagnetism*; Helsinki University of Technology: Espoo, Finland, 2001; pp. 121–124.
21. Nishimura, T.; Sakaguchi, T.; Nakagawa, S.; Hosoi, H.; Watanabe, Y.; Tonoike, M.; Imaizumi, S. Dynamic range for bone conduction ultrasound. In *Proceedings of the 12th International Conference on Biomagnetism*; Helsinki University of Technology: Espoo, Finland, 2001; pp. 125–128.
22. Nishimura, T.; Nakagawa, S.; Sakaguchi, T.; Hosoi, H.; Tonoike, M. Effect of stimulus duration for bone-conducted ultrasound on N1m in man. *Neurosci. Lett.* **2002**, *327*, 119–122. [CrossRef]
23. Yamashita, A.; Nishimura, T.; Nakagawa, S.; Sakaguchi, T.; Hosoi, H. Assessment of ability to discriminate frequency of bone-conducted ultrasound by mismatch fields. *Neurosci. Lett.* **2008**, *438*, 260–262. [CrossRef]
24. Nishimura, T.; Nakagawa, S.; Yamashita, A.; Sakaguchi, T.; Hosoi, H. N1m amplitude growth function for bone-conducted ultrasound. *Acta Otolaryngol. Suppl.* **2009**, *562*, 28–33. [CrossRef] [PubMed]
25. Okayasu, T.; Nishimura, T.; Uratani, Y.; Yamashita, A.; Nakagawa, S.; Yamanaka, T.; Hosoi, H.; Kitahara, T. Temporal window of integration estimated by omission in bone-conducted ultrasound. *Neurosci. Lett.* **2019**, *696*, 1–6. [CrossRef]
26. Dhanasingh, A.; Jolly, C. An Overview of Cochlear Implant Electrode Array Designs. *Hear. Res.* **2017**, *356*, 93–103. [CrossRef] [PubMed]
27. McRackan, T.R.; Bauschard, M.; Hatch, J.L.; Franko-Tobin, E.; Droghini, H.R.; Nguyen, S.A.; Dubno, J.R. Meta-Analysis of Quality-of-Life Improvement after Cochlear Implantation and Associations with Speech Recognition Abilities. *Laryngoscope* **2018**, *128*, 982–990. [CrossRef] [PubMed]
28. Berg, K.A.; Noble, J.H.; Dawant, B.M.; Dwyer, R.T.; Labadie, R.F.; Gifford, R.H. Speech recognition as a function of the number of channels in perimodiolar electrode recipients. *J. Acoust. Soc. Am.* **2019**, *145*, 1556–1564. [CrossRef] [PubMed]
29. Stone, M.A.; Prendergast, G.; Canavan, S. Measuring access to high-modulation-rate envelope speech cues in clinically fitted auditory prostheses. *J. Acoust. Soc. Am.* **2020**, *147*, 1284. [CrossRef]
30. Warnecke, M.; Peng, Z.E.; Litovsky, R.Y. The impact of temporal fine structure and signal envelope on auditory motion perception. *PLoS ONE.* **2020**, *15*, e0238125. [CrossRef] [PubMed]
31. Okamoto, Y.; Nakagawa, S.; Fujimoto, K.; Tonoike, M. Intelligibility of bone-conducted ultrasonic speech. *Hear. Res.* **2005**, *208*, 107–113. [CrossRef]
32. Yamashita, A.; Nishimura, T.; Nagatani, Y.; Okayasu, T.; Koizumi, T.; Sakaguchi, T.; Hosoi, H. Comparison between bone-conducted ultrasound and audible sound in speech recognition. *Acta Otolaryngol. Suppl.* **2009**, *562*, 34–39. [CrossRef] [PubMed]

33. Yamashita, A.; Nishimura, T.; Nagatani, Y.; Sakaguchi, T.; Okayasu, T.; Yanai, S.; Hosoi, H. The effect of visual information in speech signals by bone-conducted ultrasound. *NeuroReport* **2009**, *21*, 119–122. [CrossRef]
34. Dobie, R.A.; Wiederhold, M.L. Ultrasonic hearing. *Science* **1992**, *255*, 1584–1585. [CrossRef] [PubMed]
35. Fujimoto, K.; Nakagawa, S.; Tonoike, M. Nonlinear explanation for bone-conducted ultrasonic hearing. *Hear. Res.* **2005**, *204*, 210–215. [CrossRef] [PubMed]
36. Kagomiya, T.; Nakagawa, S. An evaluation of bone-conducted ultrasonic hearing-aid regarding transmission of Japanese prosodic phonemes. In *Proceedings of 20th International Congress on Acoustics*; ICA: Sydney, Australia, 2010; pp. 23–27.
37. Okayasu, T.; Nishimura, T.; Nakagawa, S.; Yamashita, A.; Nagatani, Y.; Uratani, Y.; Yamanaka, T.; Hosoi, H. Evaluation of prosodic and segmental change in speech-modulated bone-conducted ultrasound by mismatch fields. *Neurosci. Lett.* **2014**, *559*, 117–121. [CrossRef]
38. Okayasu, T.; Nishimura, T.; Yamashita, A.; Nakagawa, S.; Nagatani, Y.; Yanai, S.; Uratani, Y.; Hosoi, H. Duration-dependent growth of N1m for speech-modulated bone-conducted ultrasound. *Neurosci. Lett.* **2011**, *495*, 72–76. [CrossRef] [PubMed]
39. Nishimura, T.; Okayasu, T.; Saito, O.; Shimokura, R.; Yamashita, A.; Yamanaka, T.; Hosoi, H.; Kitahara, T. An examination of the effects of broadband air-conduction masker on the speech intelligibility of speech-modulated bone-conduction ultrasound. *Hear. Res.* **2014**, *317*, 41–49. [CrossRef] [PubMed]
40. McCormack, A.; Edmondson-Jones, M.; Somerset, S.; Hall, D. A systematic review of the reporting of tinnitus prevalence and severity. *Hear. Res.* **2016**, *337*, 70–79. [CrossRef]
41. Szibor, A.; Mäkitie, A.; Aarnisalo, A.A. Tinnitus and suicide: An unresolved relation. *Audiol. Res.* **2019**, *9*, 222. [CrossRef]
42. Ziai, K.; Moshtaghi, O.; Mahboubi, H.; Djalilian, H.R. Tinnitus patients suffering from anxiety and depression: A review. *Int. Tinnitus J.* **2017**, *21*, 68–73. [CrossRef]
43. Tinnitus Retraining Therapy Trial Research Group; Scherer, R.W.; Formby, C. Effect of Tinnitus Retraining Therapy vs Standard of Care on Tinnitus-Related Quality of Life: A Randomized Clinical Trial. *JAMA Otolaryngol. Head Neck Surg.* **2019**, *145*, 597–608. [CrossRef] [PubMed]
44. Ogawa, K.; Sato, H.; Takahashi, M.; Wada, T.; Naito, Y.; Kawase, T.; Murakami, S.; Hara, A.; Kanzaki, S. Clinical practice guidelines for diagnosis and treatment of chronic tinnitus in Japan. *Auris Nasus Larynx* **2020**, *47*, 1–6. [CrossRef]
45. Nagaraj, M.K.; Prabhu, P. Internet/smartphone-based applications for the treatment of tinnitus: A systematic review. *Eur. Arch. Otorhinolaryngol.* **2020**, *277*, 649–657. [CrossRef] [PubMed]
46. Roberts, L.E.; Moffat, G.; Bosnyak, D.J. Residual inhibition functions in relation to tinnitus spectra auditory threshold shift. *Acta Otolaryngol. Suppl.* **2006**, *556*, 27–33. [CrossRef] [PubMed]
47. Goldstein, B.A.; Lenhardt, M.L.; Shulman, A. Tinnitus improvement with ultra high frequency vibration therapy. *Int. Tinnitus J.* **2005**, *11*, 14–22.
48. Goldstein, B.A.; Shulman, A.; Lenhardt, M.L. Ultra-high frequency ultrasonic external acoustic stimulation for tinnitus relief: A method for patient selection. *Int. Tinnitus J.* **2005**, *11*, 111–114. [PubMed]
49. Koizumi, T.; Nishimura, T.; Yamashita, A.; Yamanaka, T.; Imamura, T.; Hosoi, H. Residual inhibition of tinnitus induced by 30-kHz bone-conducted ultrasound. *Hear. Res.* **2014**, *310*, 48–53. [CrossRef]

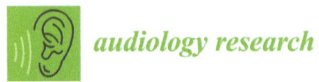

Article

Word Categorization of Vowel Durational Changes in Speech-Modulated Bone-Conducted Ultrasound

Tadao Okayasu [1,*], Tadashi Nishimura [1], Akinori Yamashita [1], Yoshiki Nagatani [2], Takashi Inoue [3], Yuka Uratani [1], Toshiaki Yamanaka [1], Hiroshi Hosoi [4] and Tadashi Kitahara [1]

[1] Department of Otolaryngology-Head and Neck Surgery, Nara Medical University, 840 Shijo-cho, Kashihara 634-8522, Japan; t-nishim@naramed-u.ac.jp (T.N.); akinori@naramed-u.ac.jp (A.Y.); ysd811yk@yahoo.co.jp (Y.U.); toshya@naramed-u.ac.jp (T.Y.); tkitahara@naramed-u.ac.jp (T.K.)
[2] Pixie Dust Technologies, 3F, 4F, Sumitomo Fudosan Suidobashi Nisiguchi Bldg, 2-20-5, Kanda-Misakicho, Chiyoda-ku, Tokyo 101-0061, Japan; yoshiki.nagatani@pixiedusttech.com
[3] Institute for Clinical and Translational Science, Nara Medical Univesity, 840 Shijo-cho, Kashihara 634-8522, Japan; tk-inoue@naramed-u.ac.jp
[4] MBT (Medicine-Based Town) Institute, Nara Medical University, 840 Shijo-cho, Kashihara 634-8522, Japan; hosoi@naramed-u.ac.jp
* Correspondence: tokayasu@naramed-u.ac.jp; Tel.: +81-744223051

Abstract: Ultrasound can deliver speech information when it is amplitude-modulated with speech and presented via bone conduction. This speech-modulated bone-conducted ultrasound (SM-BCU) can also transmit prosodic information. However, there is insufficient research on the recognition of vowel duration in SM-BCU. The aim of this study was to investigate the categorization of vowel durational changes in SM-BCU using a behavioral test. Eight Japanese-speaking participants with normal hearing participated in a forced-choice behavioral task to discriminate between "hato" (pigeon) and "haato" (heart). Speech signal stimuli were presented in seven duration grades from 220 ms to 340 ms. The threshold at which 50% of responses were "haato" was calculated and compared for air-conducted audible sound (ACAS) and SM-BCU. The boundary width was also evaluated. Although the SM-BCU threshold (mean: 274.6 ms) was significantly longer than the ACAS threshold (mean: 269.6 ms), there were no differences in boundary width. These results suggest that SM-BCU can deliver prosodic information about vowel duration with a similar difference limen to that of ACAS in normal hearing.

Keywords: bone-conduction; ultrasound; ultrasonic perception; prosody; amplitude modulation; vowel

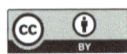

1. Introduction

Ultrasound of frequencies higher than approximately 20–24 kHz [1] are not audible to humans via air-conduction. However, when it is presented via bone-conduction, humans can perceive ultrasound up to approximately 120 kHz [2] as an auditory sensation. This phenomenon was first reported by Gavreau in 1948 [3]. Several studies have identified the characteristics of ultrasonic perception. For example, the pitch of bone-conducted ultrasound (BCU) is similar to that of high frequency air-conducted audible sound (ACAS) (approximately 8–16 kHz) [2,4,5], but the just noticeable frequency difference is worse than that of ACAS [6,7]. BCU has a narrower dynamic range of loudness than ACAS [8,9] and is difficult to mask with ACAS [4]. An interesting characteristic of BCU is that some patients with profound hearing loss can perceive BCU as an auditory sensation [6,10,11]. There are several differences in the perceptual characteristics between BCU and ACAS.

The peripheral perceptual mechanism of BCU has been studied using electrophysiological examination. One study obtained the BCU-evoked action potential using electrocochleography in guinea pigs [12]. Several studies have investigated the central perceptual mechanism of BCU in humans using magnetoencephalography (MEG) and positron-emission tomography (PET) [13–18]. Responses evoked by BCU have been detected in the auditory cortex of both normal hearing and deaf individuals [10,11]. These objective observations demonstrate that BCU is perceived as an auditory sensation.

To clarify the peripheral perceptual mechanism for BCU, the masking produced by BCU and ACAS have been investigated [8,19]. Furthermore, the impact of cisplatin administration on the BCU threshold has been evaluated in patients with head and neck cancer [20]. The results of these studies indicate the following unique peripheral perceptual mechanism of BCU. BCU perception depends on inner hair cell activity induced by ultrasound, not on enhancement by outer hair cells in the basal turn of the cochlea [8,19–21]. However, further evidence is needed to confirm this mechanism.

Some patients with profound hearing loss can hear BCU, and speech-modulated (SM) BCU can deliver speech sounds [6]. These characteristics suggest that BCU hearing aids [22] and tinnitus treatments [23] could be developed for patients with profound hearing loss. The present BCU hearing aid enables normal hearing and profoundly deaf individuals to recognize 60–70% and approximately 30% of speech words, respectively [24–27]. Moreover, prosody is important for speech information such as questions or affirmations, and for emotional expression. We demonstrated that BCU can transmit prosodic information about pitch intonation [28]. One feature of prosody is vowel duration, which plays an important role in the determination of semantic meaning in Japanese. For example, "tori" and "toori" (short- and long-duration vowels) mean bird and street, respectively. However, there is insufficient research on prosodic information about vowel duration in BCU. The aim of the present study was to investigate the categorization of vowel durational changes in SM-BCU. Assessing the ability to discriminate vowel durational changes in SM-BCU is important for the clinical application of BCU hearing aids.

2. Materials and Methods

2.1. Participants

Participants were eight healthy volunteers with normal hearing (four women, four men; age range 22–36 years). Their thresholds as determined by conventional audiometry were 20 dB HL or lower. Participants provided written consent after receiving information about all experimental procedures and the study aim. All procedures were approved by the ethics committee of Nara Medical University.

2.2. Stimuli

The categorization of "hato" or "haato" was investigated. The Japanese word "hato" has a short-duration vowel and means pigeon. The Japanese word "haato" has a long-duration vowel and means heart. The words are differentiated by the duration of the vowel /a/. Stimuli were generated based on the speech signal "hato" recorded from a native adult male in an anechoic chamber. The shortest vowel duration of /a/ in "hato" (220 ms) was extended by seven grades in 20 ms steps to produce "haato," which had the longest vowel duration (340 ms) (Figure 1). An analysis-by-synthesis system by Praat Software [29] was used to synthesize vowel duration. During editing, the same silent interval (40 ms) and syllable /to/ (90 ms) were spliced for all stimuli. The intensity and the vocal pitch contour (F0 contour) were kept constant across stimuli. The high frequency component (over 9 kHz) of the speech signal was eliminated using a low pass filter to prevent demodulation by amplitude modulation.

2.3. Discrimination Task

Participants performed a behavioral perceptual categorization task, in which they were forced to categorize stimuli as "hato" or "haato." One session consisted of 10 stimuli with seven durational grades, from 220 ms to 340 ms, in random order. The stimulus interval was set at 2.0 s. Each participant performed for a total of 70-words per presentation. The ACAS experiment was administered first, followed by the SM-BCU experiment.

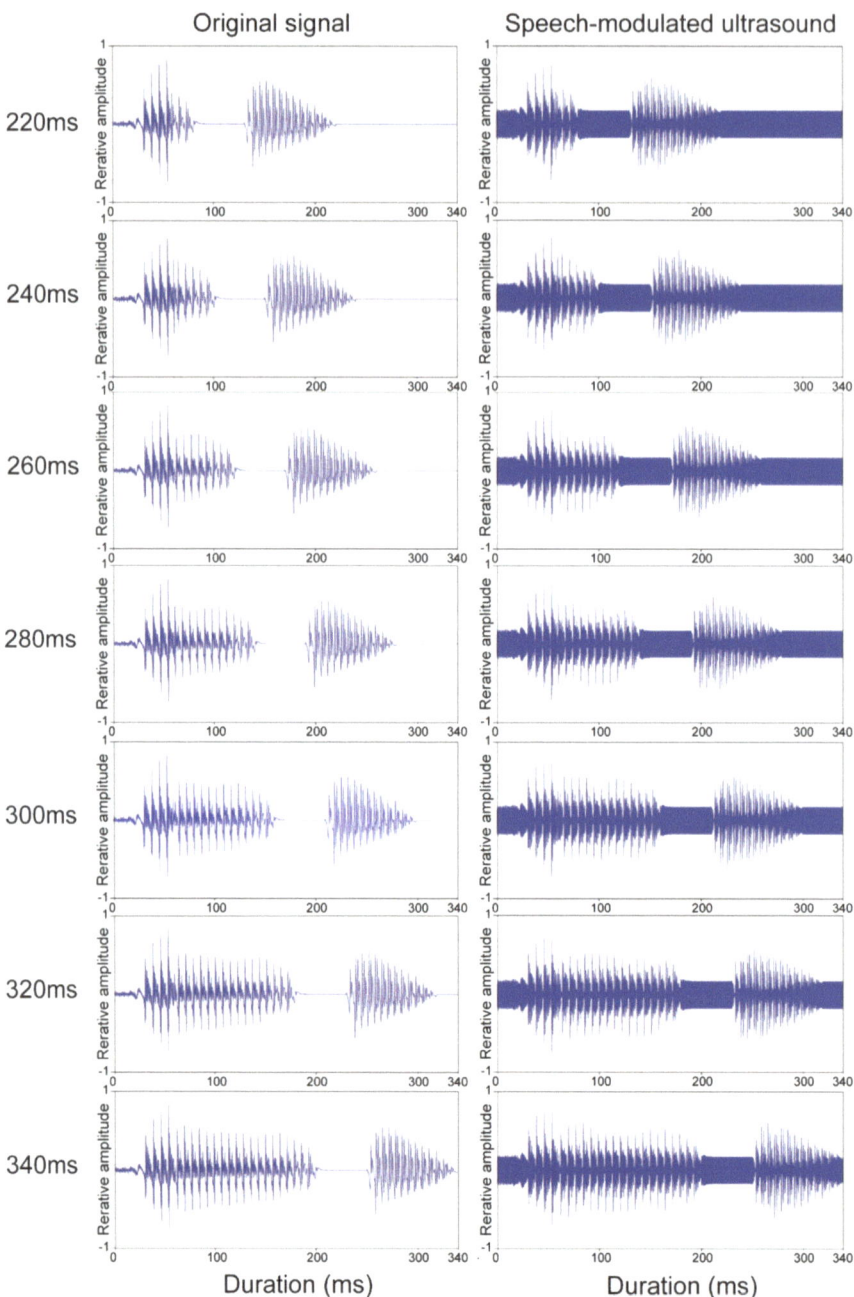

Figure 1. Speech signal waveforms of the original speech and the speech-modulated ultrasonic sounds.

2.4. Procedure

The ACAS stimuli were presented with an earphone (SR-303; STAX, Miyoshi-machi, Japan) to the left ear. The SM-BCU stimuli were presented to the left mastoid by a ceramic vibrator developed for and used in our previous study [8].

Prior to the behavioral tests, ACAS and SM-BCU thresholds for the left ear were measured for each participant using tone bursts of 1000 Hz and 30 kHz, respectively. Their duration was set to 300 ms with 50 ms rise and fall ramps. The stimulus rate was 2 Hz. ACAS and ultrasound were generated using a function generator (WF1946; NF Electronic Instruments Co., Yokohama, Japan). Sound intensities were controlled using a programmable attenuator (PA5; Tucker-Davis Technologies, Gainesville, FL, USA) with 5.0 dB and 1.0 dB steps, respectively. The obtained thresholds were operationally defined as 0 dB sensation level (SL). The ACAS test stimuli were delivered to the left ear with an intensity of 40 dB SL. The SM-BCU intensity was set at 15 dB SL to take account of the narrow dynamic range of BCU [8]. These experiments were carried out in a soundproofed room.

In the SM-BCU test, the speech stimuli were modulated onto an ultrasonic carrier with a 30 kHz sine wave. Amplitude modulation was based on a double-sideband transmitted carrier with a modulation depth of 1.0. The modulated signal was calculated using the following formula:

$$U(t) = 1/2 \times (1 + S(t)/Sc) \times \sin(2\pi f c t)$$

where S(t) is the speech signal, Sc is the peak amplitude of the sinusoidal wave whose equivalent continuous A-weighted sound pressure level was equal to the speech signals, and fc is the carrier frequency (30 kHz). Figure 1 shows the waveforms of the signals.

2.5. Analysis

To evaluate the categorization boundary, the relationship between the proportion of responses and the stimulus duration was approximated using a three-parameter logistic function. The stimulus duration at which 50% of responses were "haato" was defined as the threshold (Figure 2). The boundary width was defined as the stimulus duration at which 75% of responses were "haato" minus the stimulus duration at which 25% of responses were "haato" [30,31]. The threshold and the boundary width for ACAS and SM-BCU were calculated. These analyses were performed using JMP Pro version 15.2.1 (SAS Institute Inc., Cary, NC, USA).

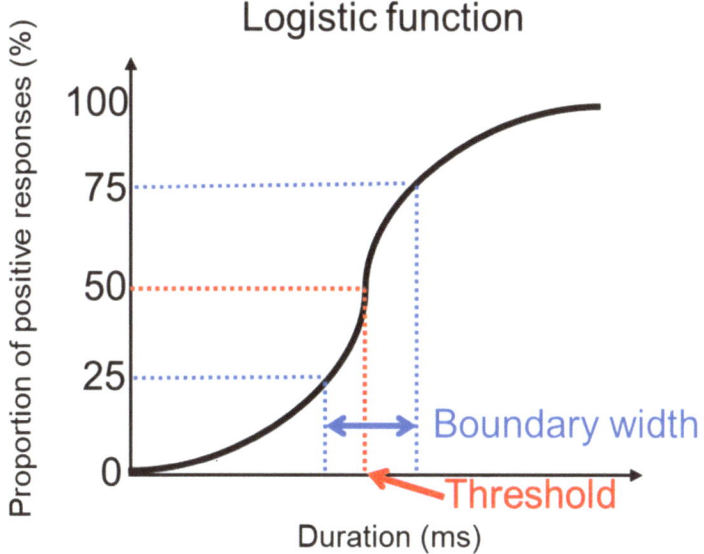

Figure 2. Evaluation of the categorization boundary using a logistic function.

2.6. Statistics

The threshold and boundary width were compared between ACAS and SM-BCU using the Wilcoxon matched-pairs signed rank test. These statistical analyses were performed using GraphPad software (GraphPad Prism version 7.02; GraphPad Software, Inc., LaJolla, CA, USA). Values of $p < 0.05$ were considered significant.

3. Results

Subjective perception of hearing for SM-BCU is an important clue for the discrimination. These participants could perceive carrier-like and speech-like sounds from SM-BCU. Even if SM-BCU, all participants could recognize the words of "hato" with the duration 220 ms at the accuracy rate of 100% and "haato" with the duration 340 ms at the accuracy rate of 95–100%. Figure 3 shows the logistic functions obtained in the behavioral tests. The threshold means for both ACAS (269.4 ms) and SM-BCU (274.6 ms) were between 260 and 280 ms. There was a significant difference between ACAS and SM-BCU thresholds ($p < 0.05$) (Figure 4a).

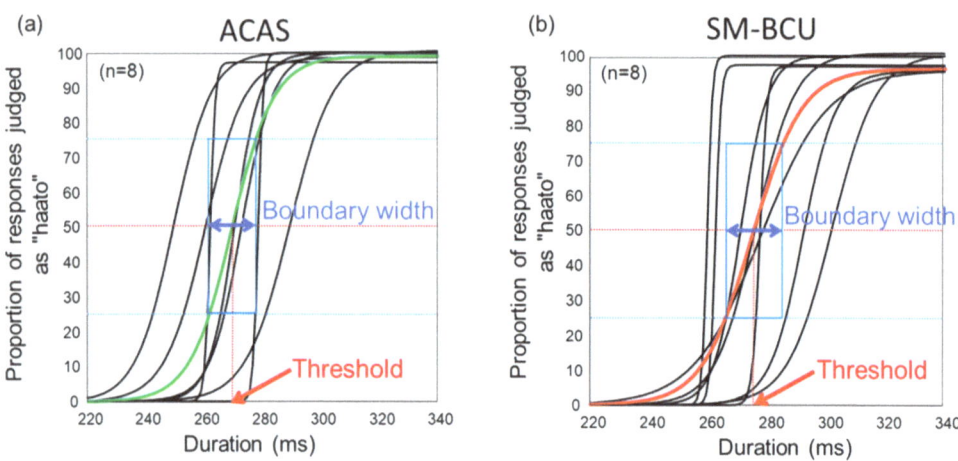

Figure 3. Logistic functions for air-conducted audible sound (ACAS) (**a**) and speech-modulated bone-conducted ultrasound (SM-BCU) (**b**).

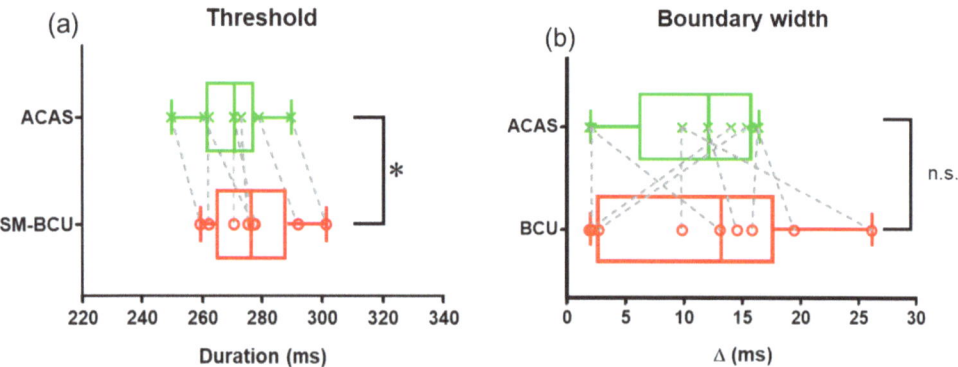

Figure 4. Threshold (**a**) and boundary width (**b**) for ACAS and SM-BCU. The asterisk indicates a statistically significant result from the Wilcoxon matched-pairs signed rank test (* $p < 0.05$). ACAS, air-conducted audible sound; SM-BCU, speech-modulated bone-conducted ultrasound.

Figure 4b shows the boundary width. There was no significant difference in boundary width between ACAS and SM-BCU ($p = 0.46$).

4. Discussion

The present study investigated the categorization boundary of vowel durational changes in SM-BCU. Although there was no difference in boundary width for the categorization of "hato" and "haato," the SM-BCU threshold was significantly longer than the ACAS threshold. These results suggest that SM-BCU can deliver prosodic information about vowel duration, and that individuals with normal hearing can categorize short- and long-duration vowels in SM-BCU with a similar difference limen to that of ACAS. The recognition of "haato" in SM-BCU required a longer-duration vowel for the categorization than in ACAS. This may be explained by the difference between SM-BCU and ACAS waveforms. Since the modulation method in this experiment was based on a double-sideband transmitted carrier, the SM-BCU waveform contained the carrier signals at the frequency of 30 kHz. The carrier signal presented consistently is a possible factor that caused the difference. Although ACAS showed silent intervals (40 ms) between the first and second syllables, the same interval in SM-BCU was occupied by the carrier signal (Figure 1). Temporal fine structure (rapid oscillations with a rate close to the central frequency of the band) plays an important role in understanding speech sounds, especially in background noise conditions [32]. Because the tail fluctuation of the envelope /ha/ in SM-BCU was unclear compared with that in ACAS (Figure 5), identification of "haato" in SM-BCU may need the longer-duration vowel. To confirm the effects of these factors, further study using other modulation methods or modulation depth is needed.

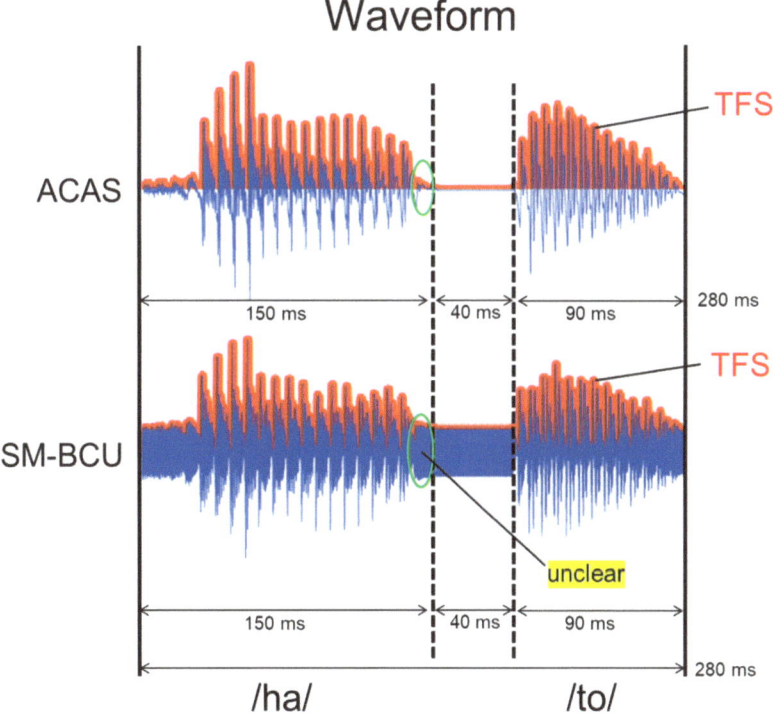

Figure 5. Envelope of 280 ms speech signal for ACAS and SM-BCU. ACAS, air-conducted audible sound; SM-BCU, speech-modulated bone-conducted ultrasound; TFS, temporal fine structure.

Findings from a previous study on the perceptual mechanism of SM-BCU in normal hearing individuals suggest that both demodulated low frequency sound and direct ultrasonic stimulation contribute to the recognition of SM-BCU [33]. Therefore, Future studies including a demodulated sound masking condition or examination for the performance of profoundly deaf individuals is needed on vowel durational changes in SM-BCU.

5. Study Limitations

This study has some limitations. We investigated word categorization of vowel durational changes for SM-BCU using only "hato" and "haato". However, in the investigation using other vowels, duration was not confirmed. Second, the effect of order in which the measurement was performed for ACAS first and followed by the SM-BCU was not counterbalanced. Third, amount of data was relatively small. Further studies are needed to prove the consistency in other vowels and words.

In summary, through the behavioral study, the evidence for the categorization of vowel durational changes was demonstrated even for SM-BCU. This study suggests that SM-BCU can deliver prosodic information about vowel duration with a similar difference limen to that of ACAS.

Author Contributions: Conceptualization, T.O., T.N., and A.Y.; methodology, T.O., Y.U., and Y.N.; behavioral examination, T.O., A.Y., and Y.U.; data analysis, T.O. and T.I.; writing—original draft preparation, T.O. and T.N.; writing—review, T.Y., H.H., and T.K.; supervision, T.K.; project administration, T.N. and H.H.; funding acquisition, T.O. All authors have read and agreed to the published version of the manuscript.

Funding: This study was supported by Grant-in-Aid for Young Scientists (B) (grant number 16K20272) and Grant-in-Aid for Scientific Research (C) (grant number 121K09588) from the Japan Society for the Promotion of Science.

Institutional Review Board Statement: This study was by the Ethics Committee of the Nara Medical University.

Informed Consent Statement: Informed consent was obtained from all subjects involved in the study.

Data Availability Statement: Not applicable.

Acknowledgments: The authors thank Takayuki Kagomiya for advice about the experiment.

Conflicts of Interest: All authors declare no conflict of interest related to this manuscript.

References

1. Wegel, R.P. Physical data and physiology of excitation of the auditory nerve. *Ann. Otol. Rhinol. Laryngol.* **1932**, *41*, 740–799. [CrossRef]
2. Pumphrey, R. Upper limit of frequency for human hearing. *Nature* **1950**, *166*, 571. [CrossRef]
3. Gavreau, V. Audibillite de sons de frequence elevee. *C. R.* **1948**, *226*, 2053–2054.
4. Dieroff, H.G.; Ertel, H. Some thoughts on the perception of ultrasound by man. *Arch. Otorhinolaryngol.* **1975**, *209*, 277–290. [CrossRef]
5. Haeff, A.V.; Knox, C. Perception of ultrasound. *Science* **1963**, *139*, 590–592. [CrossRef]
6. Lenhardt, M.L.; Skellett, R.; Wang, P.; Clarke, A.M. Human ultrasonic speech perception. *Science* **1991**, *253*, 82–85. [CrossRef]
7. Yamashita, A.; Nishimura, T.; Nakagawa, S.; Sakaguchi, T.; Hosoi, H. Assessment of ability to discriminate frequency of bone-conducted ultrasound by mismatch fields. *Neurosci. Lett.* **2008**, *438*, 260–262.
8. Nishimura, T.; Nakagawa, S.; Sakaguchi, T.; Hosoi, H. Ultrasonic masker clarifies ultrasonic perception in man. *Hear. Res.* **2003**, *175*, 171–177. [CrossRef]
9. Nishimura, T.; Nakagawa, S.; Yamashita, A.; Sakaguchi, T.; Hosoi, H. N1m amplitude growth function for bone-conducted ultrasound. *Acta Otolaryngol. Suppl.* **2009**, *562*, 28–33. [CrossRef]
10. Hosoi, H.; Imaizumi, S.; Sakaguchi, T.; Tonoike, M.; Murata, K. Activation of the auditory cortex by ultrasound. *Lancet* **1998**, *351*, 496–497. [CrossRef]
11. Imaizumi, S.; Mori, K.; Kiritani, S.; Hosoi, H.; Tonoike, M. Task-dependent laterality for cue decoding during spoken language processing. *Neuroreport* **1998**, *30*, 899–903. [CrossRef]
12. Ohyama, K.; Kusakari, J.; Kawamoto, K. Ultrasonic electrocochleography in guinea pig. *Hear. Res.* **1985**, *17*, 143–151. [CrossRef]

13. Nishimura, T.; Sakaguchi, T.; Nakagawa, S.; Hosoi, H.; Watanabe, Y.; Tonoike, M.; Imaizumi, S. Dynamic range for bone conduction ultrasound. In Proceedings of the 12th International Conference on Biomagnetism, Espoo, Finland, 13–17 August 2000; pp. 125–128.
14. Sakaguchi, T.; Hirano, T.; Nishimura, T.; Nakagawa, S.; Watanabe, Y.; Hosoi, H.; Imaizumi, S.; Tonoike, M. Cerebral neuromagnetic responses evoked by two-channel bone-conducted ultrasound stimuli. In Proceedings of the 12th International Conference on Biomagnetism, Espoo, Finland, 13–17 August 2000; pp. 121–124.
15. Nishimura, T.; Nakagawa, S.; Sakaguchi, T.; Hosoi, H.; Tonoike, M. Effect of stimulus duration for bone-conducted ultrasound on N1m in man. *Neurosci. Lett.* **2002**, *327*, 119–122. [CrossRef]
16. Sakaguchi, T.; Hirano, T.; Watanabe, Y.; Nishimura, T.; Hosoi, H.; Imaizumi, S.; Nakagawa, S.; Tonoike, M. Inner head acoustic field for bone-conducted sound calculated by finite-difference time-domain method. *Jpn. J. Appl. Phys.* **2002**, *41*, 3604–3608. [CrossRef]
17. Okayasu, T.; Nishimura, T.; Yamashita, A.; Nakagawa, S.; Nagatani, Y.; Yanai, S.; Uratani, Y.; Hosoi, H. Duration-dependent growth of N1m for speech-modulated bone-conducted ultrasound. *Neurosci. Lett.* **2011**, *495*, 72–76. [CrossRef]
18. Okayasu, T.; Nishimura, T.; Uratani, Y.; Yamashita, A.; Nakagawa, S.; Yamanaka, T.; Hosoi, H.; Kitahara, T. Temporal window of integration estimated by omission in bone-conducted ultrasound. *Neurosci. Lett.* **2019**, *696*, 1–6. [CrossRef]
19. Nishimura, T.; Okayasu, T.; Uratani, Y.; Fukuda, F.; Saito, O.; Hosoi, H. Peripheral perception mechanism of ultrasonic hearing. *Hear. Res.* **2011**, *277*, 176–183. [CrossRef]
20. Okayasu, T.; Nishimura, T.; Yamashita, A.; Saito, O.; Fukuda, F.; Yanai, S.; Hosoi, H. Human ultrasonic hearing is induced by a direct ultrasonic stimulation of the cochlea. *Neurosci. Lett.* **2013**, *539*, 71–76.
21. Nishimura, T.; Okayasu, T.; Yamashita, A.; Hosoi, H.; Kitahara, T. Perception mechanism of bone conducted ultrasound and its clinical use. *Audiol. Res.* **2021**, *11*, 244–253. [CrossRef]
22. Nakagawa, S.; Okamoto, Y.; Fujisaka, Y. Development of a bone-conducted ultrasonic hearing aid for the profoundly deaf. *Trans. Jpn. Soc. Med. Biol. Eng.* **2006**, *44*, 184–189.
23. Koizumi, T.; Nishimura, T.; Yamashita, A.; Yamanaka, T.; Imamura, T.; Hosoi, H. Residual inhibition of tinnitus induced by 30-kHz bone-conducted ultrasound. *Hear. Res.* **2014**, *310*, 48–53. [CrossRef]
24. Okamoto, Y.; Nakagawa, S.; Fujimoto, K.; Tonoike, M. Intelligibility of boneconducted ultrasonic speech. *Hear. Res.* **2005**, *208*, 107–113. [CrossRef]
25. Yamashita, A.; Nishimura, T.; Nagatani, Y.; Okayasu, T.; Koizumi, T.; Sakaguchi, T.; Hosoi, H. Comparison between bone-conducted ultrasound and audible sound in speech recognition. *Acta Otolaryngol. Suppl.* **2009**, *562*, 34–39. [CrossRef]
26. Yamashita, A.; Nishimura, T.; Nagatani, Y.; Sakaguchi, T.; Okayasu, T.; Yanai, S.; Hosoi, H. The effect of visual information in speech signals by bone-conducted ultrasound. *Neuroreport* **2009**, *21*, 119–122. [CrossRef]
27. Shimokura, R.; Fukuda, F.; Hosoi, H. A case study of auditory rehabilitation in a deaf participant using a bone-conducted ultrasonic hearing aid. *Behav. Sci. Res.* **2012**, *50*, 187–198.
28. Okayasu, T.; Nishimura, T.; Nakagawa, S.; Yamashita, A.; Nagatani, Y.; Uratani, Y.; Yamanaka, T.; Hosoi, H. Evaluation of prosodic and segmental change in speechmodulated bone-conducted ultrasound by mismatch fields. *Neurosci. Lett.* **2014**, *559*, 117–121.
29. Boersma, P.; Weenink, D. Praat: Doing Phonetics by Computer. Version 5.1.04. Available online: http://www.praat.org/ (accessed on 4 April 2009).
30. Levitt, H. Transformed up-down methods in psychoacoustics. *J. Acoust. Soc. Am.* **1971**, *49* (Suppl. S2), 467–477. [CrossRef]
31. Kagomiya, T.; Nakagawa, S. An evaluation of bone-conducted ultrasonic hearing-aid regarding transmission of Japanese prosodic phonemes. In Proceedings of the 20th International Congress on Acoustics, ICA, Sydney, Australia, 23–27 August 2010; pp. 23–27.
32. Lorenzi, C.; Gilbert, G.; Carn, H.; Garnier, S.; Moore, B.C. Speech perception problems of the hearing impaired reflect inability to use temporal fine structure. *Proc. Natl. Acad. Sci. USA* **2006**, *103*, 18866–18869. [CrossRef]
33. Nishimura, T.; Okayasu, T.; Saito, O.; Shimokura, R.; Yamashita, A.; Yamanaka, T.; Hosoi, H.; Kitahara, T. An examination of the effects of broadband air-conduction masker on the speech intelligibility of speech-modulated bone-conduction ultrasound. *Hear. Res.* **2014**, *317*, 41–49. [CrossRef]

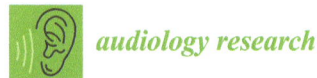

Review

Cartilage Conduction Hearing and Its Clinical Application

Tadashi Nishimura [1,*], Hiroshi Hosoi [2], Ryota Shimokura [3], Chihiro Morimoto [1] and Tadashi Kitahara [1]

1. Department of Otolaryngology-Head and Neck Surgery, Nara Medical University, 840 Shijo-cho, Kashihara, Nara 634-8522, Japan; mori-chi@naramed-u.ac.jp (C.M.); tkitahara@naramed-u.ac.jp (T.K.)
2. MBT (Medicine-Based Town) Institute, Nara Medical University, 840 Shijo-cho, Kashihara, Nara 634-8522, Japan; hosoi@naramed-u.ac.jp
3. Graduate School of Engineering Science, Osaka University, D436, 1-3 Machikaneyama, Toyonaka, Osaka 560-8531, Japan; rshimo@sys.es.osaka-u.ac.jp
* Correspondence: t-nishim@naramed-u.ac.jp; Tel.: +81-744-22-3051

Abstract: Cartilage conduction (CC) is a form of conduction that allows a relatively loud sound to be audible when a transducer is placed on the aural cartilage. The CC transmission mechanism has gradually been elucidated, allowing for the development of CC hearing aids (CC-HAs), which are clinically available in Japan. However, CC is still not fully understood. This review summarizes previous CC reports to facilitate its understanding. Concerning the transmission mechanism, the sound pressure level in the ear canal was found to increase when the transducer was attached to the aural cartilage, compared to an unattached condition. Further, inserting an earplug and injecting water into the ear canal shifted the CC threshold, indicating the considerable influence of cartilage–air conduction on the transmission. In CC, the aural cartilage resembles the movable plate of a vibration speaker. This unique transduction mechanism is responsible for the CC characteristics. In terms of clinical applications, CC-HAs are a good option for patients with aural atresia, despite inferior signal transmission compared to bone conduction in bony atretic ears. The advantages of CC, namely comfort, stable fixation, esthetics, and non-invasiveness, facilitate its clinical use.

Keywords: cartilage conduction; airborne sound; aural atresia; hearing aid; bone conduction; bone-anchored hearing aid; conductive hearing loss

Citation: Nishimura, T.; Hosoi, H.; Shimokura, R.; Morimoto, C.; Kitahara, T. Cartilage Conduction Hearing and Its Clinical Application. *Audiol. Res.* **2021**, *11*, 254–262. https://doi.org/10.3390/audiolres 11020023

Academic Editor: Tobias Neher

Received: 30 April 2021
Accepted: 1 June 2021
Published: 3 June 2021

Publisher's Note: MDPI stays neutral with regard to jurisdictional claims in published maps and institutional affiliations.

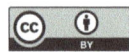

Copyright: © 2021 by the authors. Licensee MDPI, Basel, Switzerland. This article is an open access article distributed under the terms and conditions of the Creative Commons Attribution (CC BY) license (https://creativecommons.org/licenses/by/4.0/).

1. Introduction

The sound transmission pathway to the cochlea is generally classified into air and bone conduction (AC and BC). For AC, sound generated outside the ear travels to the eardrum through the ear canal and is transduced into vibrations of the ossicles to reach the cochlea. For BC, skull bone vibrations induced by a transducer are transmitted to the cochlea, involving at least five components [1–3]. Sound can also be perceived by body part vibrations other than the skull bone [4–6], and the transmission mechanisms are unique from one another. When the transducer is placed on the aural cartilage, particularly on the tragus, a relatively loud sound is audible [7]. This form of conduction is referred to as cartilage conduction (CC) [8]. Generally, hearing through non-osseous soft tissue conduction is not as clear as conventional BC. However, a clear sound is audible in CC, and it is perceived louder than when a transducer is placed on the mastoid or forehead [9].

The hypothesized CC mechanism is different from AC and BC [10,11]. For a vibration speaker, the sound signal increases by a movable plate, and the amplified signal is transmitted via AC. For CC, the vibration of the cartilaginous portion of the ear canal induced by a transducer generates sound in the ear canal. In this transduction, the cartilaginous portion of the ear canal functions like the movable plate of a vibration speaker, and thus the signal in the ear canal increases in amplitude compared to when the transducer is unattached to the aural cartilage. The airborne sound in the canal is subsequently transmitted via the eardrum in the same manner as with AC. The signal is predominately transmitted via the eardrum and ossicles, although CC delivers the signals by vibrating a transducer, similar to

BC or non-osseous BC. Therefore, the conduction characteristics resemble AC rather than BC. In contrast to AC, CC uses the aural cartilage in the same way as the moveable plate of a vibration speaker to generate airborne sound. In other words, a part of the human body (aural cartilage) contributes to airborne sound generation. This hypothesis underlying the generation of airborne sound in CC is unique and currently not fully understood. Due to the unique characteristics of CC, acoustic devices utilizing CC may potentially provide benefits that cannot be obtained with AC or BC devices. To develop CC devices further, the mechanism underlying the conduction must be established. With this review, we aim to summarize previous reports regarding CC that we found on PubMed (search term "cartilage conduction hearing") to facilitate its understanding.

2. The Theoretical CC Transmission Pathway

There are three possible transmission pathways when a transducer is placed on the aural cartilage, as presented in Figure 1 [10,11]. In the first pathway, transducer vibrations directly produce airborne sound, some of which reach the ear canal and are transmitted to the cochlea via the conventional AC pathway. This pathway is termed "direct-AC" and has the same transduction mechanism as AC. In the second pathway, aural cartilage vibrations are transmitted to the cartilaginous portion of the ear canal. These vibrations induce an acoustic signal in the canal that reaches the eardrum, transmitted via the ossicles. This pathway, which uses the aural cartilage as a movable plate, is termed "cartilage-AC" and is a transduction mechanism different from those of AC and BC. In the third pathway, aural cartilage vibrations are transmitted via the skull. This pathway is termed "cartilage-BC," and is considered similar to BC because the delivered mechanical signal is directly transmitted via the skull bone.

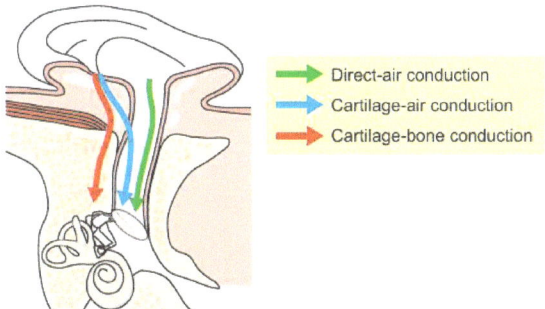

Figure 1. Possible cartilage conduction pathways. (Figure 1 was originally presented in Nishimura et al. 2015, Figure 1 [11]).

3. Sound Pressure Level in the Ear Canal via CC

A loud sound is audible when a transducer is attached to the aural cartilage. There are no standard evaluation methods for CC hearing. The measurement of the sound level in the ear canal similar to real-ear measurements [12] contributes towards understanding the phenomenon. Shimokura et al. objectively demonstrated the loudness increase by measuring the sound pressure level in the ear canal using a probe microphone (Figure 2) [13]. The sound pressure level in the ear canal improved when the transducer was attached to the aural cartilage compared to the unattached condition in all participants. The improvements from the attached condition were largest at low to mid frequencies, with gains reaching approximately 40 dB at frequencies between 500 Hz and 1000 Hz. Conversely, to reproduce the difference in the sound pressure level in the ear canal between the attached and unattached conditions, not only the bony portion of the ear canal but also the cartilaginous portion was necessary to consider [14]. The airborne sound generated by a simulated cartilaginous portion (movable plate) played an important role in the reproduction of the sound pressure level in a simulated ear canal. These findings suggest the predominance of the cartilage-AC pathway in CC in the attached condition.

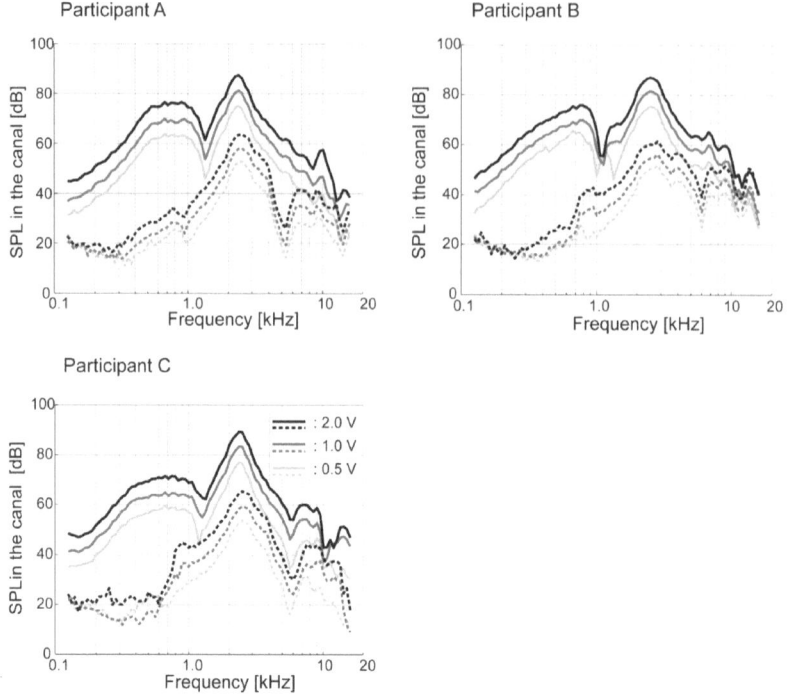

Figure 2. Sound pressure level (SPL) in the canal when the transducer is attached to the tragus (—) and unattached (- - -). The black, dark gray, and gray lines indicate input voltages of 2.0, 1.0, 0.5 V, respectively. (Figure 2 was originally presented in Shimokura et al. 2014, Figure 6 [13]).

4. Hearing Threshold Measurements via CC

4.1. Threshold Shift with an Earplug

In a previous study, an earplug was used to show differences in the characteristics between CC and AC or BC [9]. Thresholds with and without the earplug were measured at 500–4000 Hz using a transformed up-down procedure (two-alternative forced-choice) [15]. The earplug interferes with both AC and direct-AC in CC. For AC, the thresholds worsened with the earplug for all frequencies. For CC, the threshold worsened with the earplug above 2 kHz, but the thresholds at low to mid frequencies did not; they were stable at 1000 Hz and improved at 500 Hz. These observations demonstrate that direct-AC is not the predominant pathway in CC. Furthermore, for BC the thresholds at mid to high frequencies were stable with the earplug, which also disagreed with the CC results.

A transducer can be placed in various ways on the aural cartilage. Another study evaluated the effect of an earplug on the thresholds when a transducer without a static force was placed on the tragus, soft tissue (pre-tragus region), and mastoid [16]. Thresholds with and without the earplug were measured at 500–4000 Hz using a transformed up-down procedure [15]. The thresholds for the tragus placement were significantly better than for other placements, both with and without the earplug, except with the earplug at 4000 Hz. The threshold elevations with the earplug for the tragus placement were significantly larger than those for the mastoid placement at 2000 and 4000 Hz. These results demonstrate that placing the transducer on the aural cartilage contributes to hearing improvement. Low-frequency boost can influence speech perception. Although there was no deterioration in speech recognition in the open ear, excessive low-frequency boost in the occluded condition reduced the scores, even in individuals with normal hearing [17]. Frequency adjustment may be necessary for the occluded ear when excessive low-frequency boost deteriorates speech perception [18].

4.2. Threshold Shift with Water Injected into the Ear Canal

Previous studies using earplugs have contributed to establishing the conduction mechanism of CC [9,16,17]. Earplugs generate an occlusion effect, which influences low-frequency thresholds. Thus, previous studies used ear canal water injections instead of earplugs to avoid the occlusion effect [11]. AC, BC, and CC thresholds were measured at 500–4000 Hz with water injected into the ear canal using a transformed up-down procedure [15]. To measure the thresholds in the water-injected condition, subjects laid on a bed in a lateral recumbent position with the entrance of the ear canal facing the ceiling and the head fixed to avoid water fluctuations in the canal. Figure 3 illustrates the influence of water injections on three theoretical CC components. If the cartilaginous portion vibrations are dominant, the thresholds will increase when the water stays within the bony portion of the ear canal (Figure 3A), and then decrease when the water reaches the cartilaginous portion (Figure 3B). If the threshold improves when the water level is so high that it reaches the transducer (Figure 3C), then transmission through the cartilaginous portion is likely not the dominant pathway. Thus, the relationship between the threshold and water volume demonstrates the relative contribution of the three possible pathways to CC. The results of these studies revealed that injecting water into the ear canal elevated the AC thresholds by 22.6–53.3 dB, and the threshold shifts for BC were within 14.9 dB [11]. For CC, when the water was within the bony portion of the ear canal (i.e., 40% of the ear canal length in the previous study; Figure 3A), the thresholds were elevated by the same degree as AC. When the water line reached the cartilaginous portion (i.e., 80% of the ear canal length in the previous study; Figure 3B), the thresholds at 500 and 1000 Hz decreased by 27.4 and 27.5 dB, respectively. Additionally, despite blocking the ear canal with water, the force levels of the CC transducer at the thresholds measured with an artificial mastoid were clearly lower than those of the BC transducer at the threshold. The vibrations of the cartilaginous portion contributed to sound transmission, particularly in the low-frequency range. Although the airborne sound radiates into the ear canal in BC and CC, the generation mechanisms are different. CC generates airborne sounds in the canal more efficiently than BC.

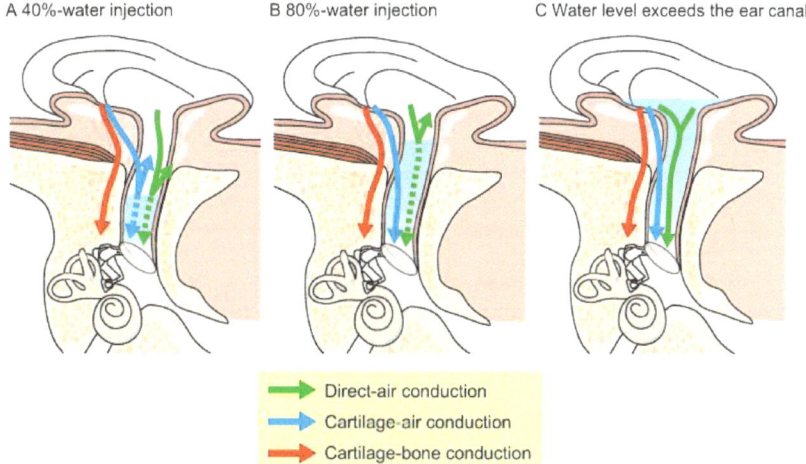

Figure 3. Effects of ear canal water injection on the transmission pathways. (**A**) The water stays within the bony portion of the ear canal, interrupting direct- and cartilage–air conduction. (**B**) The water enters the cartilaginous portion of the ear canal, avoiding an impedance mismatch between air and water in the cartilage-AC pathway. (**C**) The water level exceeds the ear canal, allowing for direct water vibrations. (Figure 3 was originally presented in Nishimura et al. 2015, Figure 1 [11]).

The effect of water in the ear canal was also evaluated at 500–2000 Hz for five different placements of the transducer: the tragus, intertragal incisure, anti-tragus, pre-tragus, and mastoid [19]. Among the CC conditions (tragus, intertragal incisure, and anti-tragus), the results showed the same amount of threshold shifts when water was injected into the ear canal, and the fixation placement did not affect the threshold shifts by water injection. Thus, the cartilage-AC characterizes the acoustic properties of CC.

5. CC in Pathological Ears

The transmission pathway or mechanism may change in pathological ears, e.g., the atretic ear whose condition is quite different from that of the normal ear. In the bony atretic ear, the AC route is not present, and most signals are transmitted to the cochlea via the skull bone. For CC, cartilage-BC is considered the predominant pathway instead of direct- and cartilage-AC (Figure 1) in the bony atretic ear. The impedance mismatch between the soft tissue and skull bone obstructs transmission. As the transducer is placed without a static force, CC and AC do not have conduction efficacy advantages over BC. Conversely, the transmission conditions in ears with fibrotic aural atresia are quite different. Vibrations are transmitted to the cochlea via fibrotic tissues instead of the skull bone. This fibrotic pathway allows the signals to travel to the cochlea, avoiding the large impedance mismatch between the soft tissue and skull bone. Some patients with fibrotic aural atresia have much better thresholds with CC (30–50 dB at low frequency compared to BC) [20]. Hence, CC has a transmission advantage over BC in the case of the fibrotic pathway.

6. CC Applications

Acoustic devices that utilize CC, including smartphones and hearing aids, have been developed [8,21–23]. CC hearing aids (HA; CC-HA) have already been used in clinical practice in Japan since 2017. When direct- and cartilage-AC are functional (such as for sensorineural hearing loss), a commercially available CC-HA (Figure 4) could provide adequate amplification for mild to moderate hearing loss, as estimated by measuring the output level using a simulator which can evaluate the airborne sound in CC [24]. When direct- and cartilage-AC are not functional, patients who receive the most benefits from CC-HAs are patients with aural atresia. These patients require BC-HAs or implantable devices to achieve sufficient amplification [25–31]. However, conventional BC-HAs have disadvantages associated with their fixation style; the transducer is fixed with a headband using static force, which can lead to discomfort, pain, and irritation [26]. The fixation of the transducer can cause poor esthetics. Surgical procedures, such as implanting bone-anchored hearing aids (BAHAs), are additional options [25–31] but involve various risks, such as adverse medical and surgical events, infection, and follow-up surgery [32,33]. Some patients also refuse BAHA implantation because of cosmetic considerations [34]. In contrast, the CC transducer is fixed without a static force, mitigating some of the fixation problems with BC-HAs, and it does not require surgery. In contrast to AC, CC mechanical signals can be delivered directly to the tissue. CC also has transmission advantages in the atretic ear over AC because it avoids the impedance mismatch between air and skin. Thus, CC-HAs are a possible alternative for patients with aural atresia.

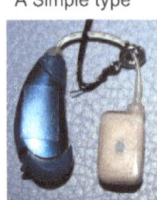
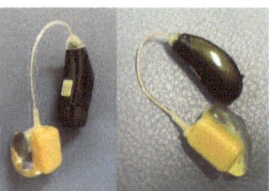
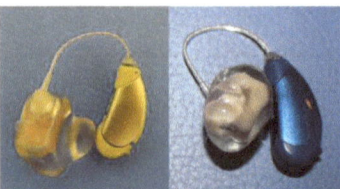

Figure 4. Cartilage conduction hearing aids (HB-J1CC, Rion Co Ltd., Kokubunji, Tokyo, Japan) have three transducer types: (**A**) simple-attachment, (**B**) ear-chip attachment, and (**C**) ear-chip embedded.

6.1. CC-HA Characteristics

CC-HAs are behind-the-ear HAs (Figure 4), with the transducer placed on the aural cartilage and the signal delivered through the cartilaginous tissue [35]. The transducer, optimized to transmit vibrations to the aural cartilage, is small and lightweight (11.9 × 7.8 × 4.7 mm, 1.4 g). It is easily attached to the ear because of the conchal cartilage stiffness, even when only a small cavity is present on the ear surface (Figure 5A). In the absence of a sufficiently large cavity, CC-HA transducers can be attached with double-sided tape (Figure 5B). Therefore, neither a high contact pressure nor a headband is required for attachment. There is little risk of skin irritation, as experienced by patients who use conventional BC-HAs, or infection, as experienced by patients with implanted BAHAs [36,37], and they can be used from infancy. In Japan, CC-HA has become an option for treating atretic ears. The Oto-Rhino-Laryngological Society of Japan puts the information related to CC hearing aids along with that related to BAHAs, Vibrant Soundbridge (VSB), and cochlea implants at its website [38], and the guidelines for implantable devices such as BAHAs, VSB and Bonebridge authorized by the Japan Otological Society [39] require CC hearing aids to be tested before the decision of their indication.

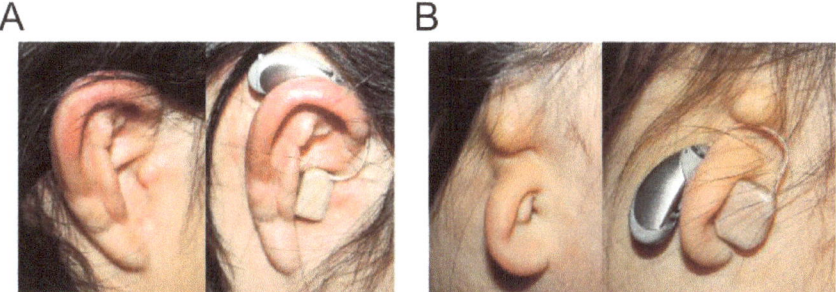

Figure 5. Examples of ears with and without cartilage conduction hearing aid (CC-HA). Some patients wear CC-HA in the same manner as conventional behind-the-ear hearing aids (**A**). For other patients, double-sided tape is needed for fixation of the hearing aids (**B**). (Figure 5 was originally presented in Nishimura et al. 2018, Figure 1 [40]).

6.2. CC-HA Benefits

CC-HAs were first reported in 2010 [21], and benefits for patients with chronic otitis media and aural atresia were reported in 2013 [22]. A clinical study with 41 patients (21 with bilateral aural atresia, 15 with unilateral aural atresia, and five with other diseases) demonstrated that CC-HAs can provide audiometric benefits equivalent to those of other devices (AC-HAs, BC-HAs, and BAHAs) without any serious adverse effects [40]. After the trial, 95% and 93% of the patients with bilateral and unilateral aural atresia, respectively, continued using their CC-HAs. Most patients who tried CC-HAs reported improvements in communication abilities in noisy environments and sound localization. Another study reported that laterality judgements significantly improved in bilateral aural atresia patients with CC-HAs [41]. Sakamoto et al. evaluated CC-HA benefits in patients with unilateral congenital atretic ears [42] and reported that speech recognition scores improved in a noisy environment. Nishiyama et al. investigated adult candidates for CC-HA treatment [43] and concluded that patients with ear canal stenosis or atretic ears were the most suited candidates. They also reported good outcomes in children with the same ear conditions [44]. To investigate the clinical use of CC-HAs in Japan, a survey was performed in nine medical institutions with 256 patients who tried CC-HAs [35]. Similar to previous studies, the survey demonstrated that the candidates for CC-HAs were patients with aural atresia. Sixty-five patients with bilaterally and 124 patients with unilaterally closed ears (aural atresia or severe canal stenosis) tried CC-HA use. The purchase rate after the trial was 86% and 78%, respectively, for these two groups of patients. Patients with refractory continuous otorrhea who experienced difficulties with AC-HA use also showed a high purchase rate (78%). In contrast, the purchase rate for patients who had no difficulty with AC-HA use, such as patients with sensorineural hearing loss, was significantly lower (37%). Finally, there were no differences between the CC-HAs and the patients' own hearing devices regarding audiometric results in the atretic ears, such as aided threshold, functional gain, and speech recognition [34,40]. Even though CC transmission is inferior to BC transmission in bony atretic ears, the audiometric outcomes were comparable [35,40], and other advantages, such as comfort, stable fixation, cosmetics, and non-invasiveness, may explain the high acceptance.

6.3. Limitations

CC-HAs have only been used in clinical practice since 2017, which is not long enough to thoroughly establish their indication criteria, fitting technique, and benefits. Furthermore, comparisons between CC-HAs and implantable devices have not been performed yet. Further investigations are therefore required for establishing CC-HAs in clinical practice.

7. Conclusions

In CC, the aural cartilage plays a similar role to the movable plate of a vibration speaker. This transduction mechanism, unique from AC and BC, is responsible for the CC characteristics. CC can be applied to various acoustic devices, and there have been rapid advances in HA development using CC. CC-HAs can be a beneficial option for patients with aural atresia, although CC does not always surpass BC in terms of transmission efficacy in bony atretic ears.

Author Contributions: Drafting the manuscript: T.N., R.S., C.M. Revising the manuscript: H.H. and T.K. Approval of the manuscript: H.H. and T.K. All authors have read and agreed to the published version of the manuscript.

Funding: This research was funded by JSPS KAKENHI, Grant Number 17K11339 and 19K09874.

Institutional Review Board Statement: Not applicable.

Informed Consent Statement: Not applicable.

Data Availability Statement: Not applicable.

Conflicts of Interest: The authors declare no conflict of interest.

References

1. Stenfelt, S.; Goode, R.L. Bone-conducted sound: Physiological and clinical aspects. *Otol. Neurotol.* **2005**, *26*, 1245–1261. [CrossRef]
2. Stenfelt, S. Acoustic and physiologic aspects of bone conduction hearing. *Adv. Otorhinolaryngol.* **2011**, *71*, 10–21. [CrossRef]
3. Stenfelt, S. Model predictions for bone conduction perception in the human. *Hear. Res.* **2016**, *340*, 135–143. [CrossRef]
4. Sohmer, H.; Freeman, S.; Geal-Dor, M.; Adelman, C.; Savion, I. Bone conduction experiments in humans—A fluid pathway from bone to ear. *Hear. Res.* **2000**, *146*, 81–88. [CrossRef]
5. Watanabe, T.; Bertoli, S.; Probst, R. Transmission pathways of vibratory stimulation as measured by subjective thresholds and distortion-product otoacoustic emissions. *Ear Hear.* **2008**, *29*, 667–673. [CrossRef] [PubMed]
6. Ito, T.; Röösli, C.; Kim, C.J.; Sim, J.H.; Huber, A.M.; Probst, R. Bone conduction thresholds and skull vibration measured on the teeth during stimulation at different sites on the human head. *Audiol. Neurootol.* **2011**, *16*, 12–22. [CrossRef]
7. Blondé-Weinmann, C.; Joubaud, T.; Zimpfer, V.; Hamery, P.; Roth, S. Characterization of cartilage implication in protected hearing perception during direct vibro-acoustic stimulation at various locations. *Appl. Acoust.* **2021**, *179*, 108074. [CrossRef]
8. Hosoi, H. Approach in the Use of Cartilage Conduction Speaker. Japanese Patent 4541111, 17 November 2004.
9. Hosoi, H.; Nishimura, T.; Shimokura, R.; Kitahara, T. Cartilage conduction as the third pathway for sound transmission. *Auris Nasus Larynx* **2019**, *46*, 151–159. [CrossRef]
10. Nishimura, T.; Hosoi, H.; Saito, O.; Miyamae, R.; Shimokura, R.; Matsui, T.; Yamanaka, T.; Levitt, H. Is cartilage conduction classified into air or bone conduction? *Laryngoscope* **2014**, *124*, 1214–1219. [CrossRef]
11. Nishimura, T.; Hosoi, H.; Saito, O.; Miyamae, R.; Shimokura, R.; Yamanaka, T.; Kitahara, T.; Levitt, H. Cartilage conduction is characterized by vibrations of the cartilaginous portion of the ear canal. *PLoS ONE* **2015**, *10*, e0120135. [CrossRef] [PubMed]
12. Gazia, F.; Galletti, B.; Portelli, D.; Alberti, G.; Freni, F.; Bruno, R.; Galletti, F. Real ear measurement (REM) and auditory performances with open, tulip and double closed dome in patients using hearing aids. *Eur. Arch. Otorhinolaryngol.* **2020**, *277*, 1289–1295. [CrossRef]

13. Shimokura, R.; Hosoi, H.; Nishimura, T.; Yamanaka, T.; Levitt, H. Cartilage conduction hearing. *J. Acoust. Soc. Am.* **2014**, *135*, 1959–1966. [CrossRef] [PubMed]
14. Shimokura, R.; Hosoi, H.; Nishimura, T.; Iwakura, T.; Yamanaka, T. Simulating cartilage conduction sound to estimate the sound pressure level in the external auditory canal. *J. Sound Vib.* **2015**, *20*, 261–268. [CrossRef]
15. Levitt, H. Transformed up-down methods in psychoacoustics. *J. Acoust. Soc. Am.* **1971**, *49*, 467–477. [CrossRef]
16. Nishimura, T.; Hosoi, H.; Saito, O.; Miyamae, R.; Shimokura, R.; Matsui, T.; Yamanaka, T.; Kitahara, T.; Levitt, H. Cartilage conduction efficiently generates airborne sound in the ear canal. *Auris Nasus Larynx* **2015**, *42*, 15–19. [CrossRef] [PubMed]
17. Miyamae, R.; Nishimura, T.; Hosoi, H.; Saito, O.; Shimokura, R.; Yamanaka, T.; Kitahara, T. Perception of speech in cartilage conduction. *Auris Nasus Larynx* **2017**, *44*, 26–32. [CrossRef] [PubMed]
18. Nishimura, T.; Miyamae, R.; Hosoi, H.; Saito, O.; Shimokura, R.; Yamanaka, T.; Kitahara, T. Frequency characteristics and speech recognition in cartilage conduction. *Auris Nasus Larynx* **2019**, *46*, 709–715. [CrossRef]
19. Nishimura, T.; Hosoi, H.; Saito, O.; Akasaka, S.; Shimokura, R.; Yamanaka, T.; Kitahara, T. Effect of fixation place on airborne sound in cartilage conduction. *J. Acoust. Soc. Am.* **2020**, *148*, 469. [CrossRef] [PubMed]
20. Morimoto, C.; Nishimura, T.; Hosoi, H.; Saito, O.; Fukuda, F.; Shimokura, R.; Yamanaka, T. Sound transmission by cartilage conduction in ear with fibrotic aural atresia. *J. Rehabil. Res. Dev.* **2014**, *51*, 325–332. [CrossRef] [PubMed]
21. Hosoi, H.; Yanai, S.; Nishimura, T.; Sakaguchi, T.; Iwakura, T.; Yoshino, K. Development of cartilage conduction hearing aid. *Arch. Mat. Sci. Eng.* **2010**, *42*, 104–110.
22. Nishimura, T.; Hosoi, H.; Saito, O.; Miyamae, R.; Shimokura, R.; Matsui, T.; Iwakura, T. Benefit of a new hearing device utilizing cartilage conduction. *Auris Nasus Larynx* **2013**, *40*, 440–446. [CrossRef] [PubMed]
23. Shimokura, R.; Hosoi, H.; Iwakura, T.; Nishimura, T.; Matsui, T. Development of monaural and binaural behind-the-ear cartilage conduction hearing aids. *Appl. Acoust.* **2013**, *74*, 1234–1240. [CrossRef]
24. Nishimura, T.; Hosoi, H.; Morimoto, C.; Kitahara, T. Indications of hearing levels for cartilage conduction hearing aids: Evaluation using 2 cm3 coupler and an artificial mastoid. *Pediatr. Otorhinolaryngol. Jpn.* **2020**, *41*, 34–40. [CrossRef]
25. House, J.W.; Kutz, J.W., Jr.; Chung, J.; Fisher, L.M. Bone-anchored hearing aid subjective benefit for unilateral deafness. *Laryngoscope* **2010**, *120*, 601–607. [CrossRef]
26. Lo, J.F.W.; Tsang, W.S.S.; Yu, J.Y.K.; Ho, O.Y.M.; Ku, P.K.M.; Tong, M.C.F. Contemporary hearing rehabilitation options in patients with aural atresia. *BioMed Res. Int.* **2014**, *2014*, 761579. [CrossRef] [PubMed]
27. Riss, D.; Arnoldner, C.; Baumgartner, W.D.; Blineder, M.; Flak, S.; Bachner, A.; Gstoettner, W.; Hamzavi, J.S. Indication criteria and outcomes with the Bonebridge transcutaneous bone-conduction implant. *Laryngoscope* **2014**, *124*, 2802–2806. [CrossRef] [PubMed]
28. Ikeda, R.; Hidaka, H.; Murata, T.; Miyazaki, H.; Katori, Y.; Kobayashi, T. Vibrant Soundbridge implantation via a retrofacial approach in a patient with congenital aural atresia. *Auris Nasus Larynx* **2019**, *46*, 204–209. [CrossRef]
29. Oh, S.J.; Goh, E.K.; Choi, S.W.; Lee, S.; Lee, H.M.; Lee, I.W.; Kong, S.K. Audiologic, surgical and subjective outcomes of active transcutaneous bone conduction implant system (Bonebridge). *Int. J. Audiol.* **2019**, *58*, 956–963. [CrossRef]
30. Curca, I.A.; Parsa, V.; Macpherson, E.A.; Scollie, S.; Vansevenant, K.; Zimmerman, K.; Lewis-Teeter, J.; Allen, P.; Parnes, L.; Agrawal, S. Audiological outcome measures with the BONEBRIDGE transcutaneous bone conduction hearing implant: Impact of noise, reverberation and signal processing features. *Int. J. Audiol.* **2020**, *59*, 556–565. [CrossRef]
31. Kwak, S.H.; Moon, Y.M.; Nam, G.S.; Bae, S.H.; Kim, S.H.; Jung, J.; Choi, J.Y. Clinical Experience of Vibroplasty With Direct Coupling to the Oval Window Without Use of a Coupler. *Laryngoscope* **2020**, *130*, E926–E932. [CrossRef]
32. Vickers, D.; Canas, A.; Degun, A.; Briggs, J.; Bingham, M.; Toner, J.; Cooper, H.; Rogers, S.; Cooper, S.; Irving, R.; et al. Evaluating the effectiveness and reliability of the Vibrant Soundbridge and Bonebridge auditory implants in clinical practice: Study design and methods for a multi-centre longitudinal observational study. *Contemp. Clin. Trials Commun.* **2018**, *10*, 137–140. [CrossRef] [PubMed]
33. Kruyt, I.J.; Bakkum, K.H.E.; Caspers, C.J.I.; Hol, M.K.S. The efficacy of bone-anchored hearing implant surgery in children: A systematic review. *Int. J. Pediatr. Otorhinolaryngol.* **2020**, *132*, 109906. [CrossRef]
34. Zawawi, F.; Kabbach, G.; Lallemand, M.; Daniel, S.J. Bone-anchored hearing aid: Why do some patients refuse it? *Int. J. Pediatr. Otorhinolaryngol.* **2014**, *78*, 232–234. [CrossRef]
35. Nishimura, T.; Hosoi, H.; Sugiuchi, T.; Matsumoto, N.; Nishiyama, T.; Takano, K.; Sugimoto, S.; Yazama, H.; Sato, T.; Komori, M. Cartilage conduction hearing aid fitting in clinical practice. *J. Am. Acad. Audiol.* **2021**, in press.
36. House, J.W.; Kutz, J.W., Jr. Bone-anchored hearing aids: Incidence and management of postoperative complications. *Otol. Neurotol.* **2007**, *28*, 213–217. [CrossRef] [PubMed]
37. Hobson, J.C.; Roper, A.J.; Andrew, R.; Rothera, M.P.; Hill, P.; Green, K.M. Complications of bone-anchored hearing aid implantation. *J. Laryngol. Otol.* **2010**, *124*, 132–136. [CrossRef] [PubMed]
38. Options for the Compensation of Hearing Loss; Different from Air and Bone Conduction Hearing Aids. Available online: http://www.jibika.or.jp/citizens/hochouki/sentaku.html (accessed on 29 April 2021).
39. Indication Criteria and Guidelines. Available online: https://www.otology.gr.jp/about/guideline.html#guideline2 (accessed on 29 April 2021).
40. Nishimura, T.; Hosoi, H.; Saito, O.; Shimokura, R.; Yamanaka, T.; Kitahara, T. Cartilage Conduction Hearing Aids for Severe Conduction Hearing Loss. *Otol. Neurotol.* **2018**, *39*, 65–72. [CrossRef]

41. Nishimura, T.; Hosoi, H.; Saito, O.; Shimokura, R.; Yamanaka, T.; Kitahara, T. Sound localisation ability using cartilage conduction hearing aids in bilateral aural atresia. *Int. J. Audiol.* **2020**, *59*, 891–896. [CrossRef]
42. Sakamoto, Y.; Shimada, A.; Nakano, S.; Kondo, E.; Takeyama, T.; Fukuda, J.; Udaka, J.; Okamoto, H.; Takeda, N. Effects of FM system fitted into the normal hearing ear or cartilage conduction hearing aid fitted into the affected ear on speech-in-noise recognition in Japanese children with unilateral congenital aural atresia. *J. Med. Investig.* **2020**, *67*, 131–138. [CrossRef]
43. Nishiyama, T.; Oishi, N.; Ogawa, K. Who are good adult candidates for cartilage conduction hearing aids? *Eur. Arch. Otorhinolaryngol.* **2020**, in press. [CrossRef]
44. Nishiyama, T.; Oishi, N.; Ogawa, K. Efficacy of cartilage conduction hearing aids in children. *Int. J. Pediatr. Otorhinolaryngol.* **2021**, *142*, 110628. [CrossRef] [PubMed]

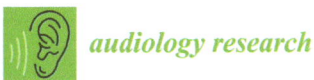

Article

Vibrational and Acoustical Characteristics of Ear Pinna Simulators That Differ in Hardness

Ryota Shimokura [1],*, Tadashi Nishimura [2] and Hiroshi Hosoi [3]

1. Department of Systems Science, Graduate School of Engineering Science, Osaka University, Osaka 560-8531, Japan
2. Department of Otolaryngology—Head & Neck Surgery, Nara Medical University, Nara 634-8521, Japan; t-nishim@naramed-u.ac.jp
3. Medicine-Based Town Institute, Nara Medical University, Nara 634-8521, Japan; hosoi@naramed-u.ac.jp
* Correspondence: rshimo@sys.es.osaka-u.ac.jp; Tel./Fax: +81-6-6850-6376

Abstract: Because cartilage conduction—the transmission of sound via the aural cartilage—has different auditory pathways from well-known air and bone conduction, how the output volume in the external auditory canal is stimulated remains unknown. To develop a simulator approximating the conduction of sound in ear cartilage, the vibrations of the pinna and sound in the external auditory canal were measured using pinna simulators made of silicon rubbers of different hardness (A40, A20, A10, A5, A0) as measured by a durometer. The same procedure, as well as a current calibration method for air conduction devices, was applied to an existing pinna simulator, the Head and Torso Simulator (hardness A5). The levels for vibration acceleration and sound pressure from these pinna simulators show spectral peaks at dominant frequencies (below 1.5 kHz) for the conduction of sound in cartilage. These peaks were likely to move to lower frequencies as hardness decreases. On approaching the hardness of actual aural cartilage (A10 to A20), the simulated levels for vibration acceleration and sound pressure approximated the measurements of human ears. The adjustment of the hardness used in pinna simulators is an important factor in simulating accurately the conduction of sound in cartilage.

Keywords: cartilage conduction; pinna simulator; head-and-torso simulator; hearing aid; vibration acceleration level; sound pressure level

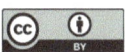

1. Introduction

Aural cartilage gives form to the pinna and the exterior half of the external auditory canal. If the aural cartilage vibrates, sound can be clearly heard [1,2]. This phenomenon is termed *cartilage conduction*, and hearing aids based on cartilage conduction [2–5] have been marketed in Japan since November 2017. When a small transducer is fixed at the entrance of the ear canal, it can generate sound via the aural cartilage into the external auditory canal (Figure 1) [6–9]. That is, this cartilage acts as a diaphragm and the transducer functions as a voice coil of a loudspeaker. Distinct from bone-conduction hearing aids, the cartilage conduction transducer is small and light, and contact pressure on the cartilage is very low because the cartilage is light and vibrates more easily than heavy skull bone. Indeed, the vibrations propagating through skull bone are small enough that their contribution to hearing can be ignored when the cartilage is stimulated [5].

Although cartilage conduction hearing aids can decrease hearing thresholds, especially of users with aural atresia, otorrhea, and microtia [10,11], they are not covered by insurance for the physically handicapped persons in Japan, because output volumes have not been standardized. Because the transmission pathway of cartilage conduction differs from either air or bone conduction (Figure 1), their calibration methods, standardized in the International Organization for Standardization [12,13], do not apply to cartilage conduction-based devices. For example, for air conduction, the sound pressure at the ear drum can be simulated using an ear simulator [14] embedded in a head-and-torso simulator (HATS) [15]. However, in terms of the cartilage sound, the HATS cannot output the same sound pressure as actual measurements from human ears, especially in the low-frequency range below 1.5 kHz [16]. Nevertheless, a soft polyurethane pipe can simulate the aural cartilage of the external auditory canal and a skull bone model can produce the sound pressure in agreement with data from human ears in this low-frequency range [13]. In that study, a ring-shaped transducer (same type in Figure 2) adhered to the pipe and was worn by seven participants, and the sound pressures in the polyurethane pipe and human canal were measured by a probe microphone, which was inserted in the pipe and canal to a point 15 mm from each entrance. The polyurethane resin was designed to simulate the elasticity of human skin (human skin gel, Exseal Corporation, Mino, Japan). In contrast, the pinna simulator of the HATS (Type 4128; Brüel & Kjaer, Naerum, Denmark) is embedded as a unit in a silicon rubber base (width × height × thickness: 50 × 60 × 10 mm^3). The hardness (Shore 00 35 or Shore A5 from durometer measurements) of the pinna simulator is lower than that of the aural cartilage of humans. In the low-frequency range, simulation results are likely to disagree because of this mismatch in hardness for the pinna simulator of HATS.

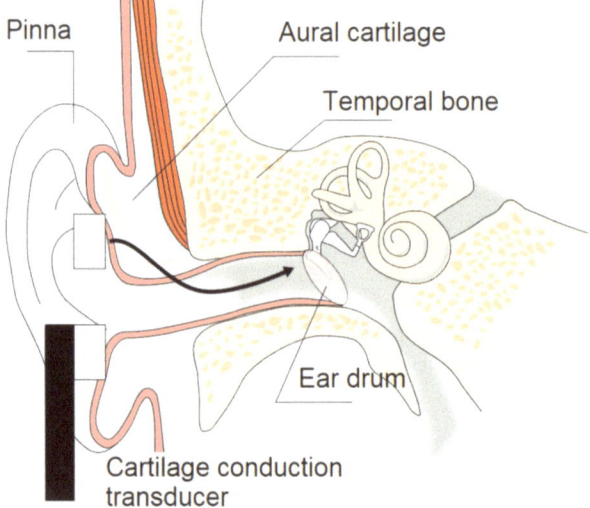

Figure 1. Cartilage conduction pathway for users without hearing impairments.

Therefore, the propagating vibration in aural cartilage and generating sound in the external auditory canal were measured in our study of five ear simulators, each made of silicon rubber of a different hardness. A hardness of aural cartilage was measured at the tragus beforehand (see Section 2.3), and the hardness of the silicon rubbers were determined to diverge higher and lower than it. For comparison, the same measurements were recorded for the pinna simulator of the HATS. Different spectral characteristics were observed that depended on the hardness of each silicon rubber.

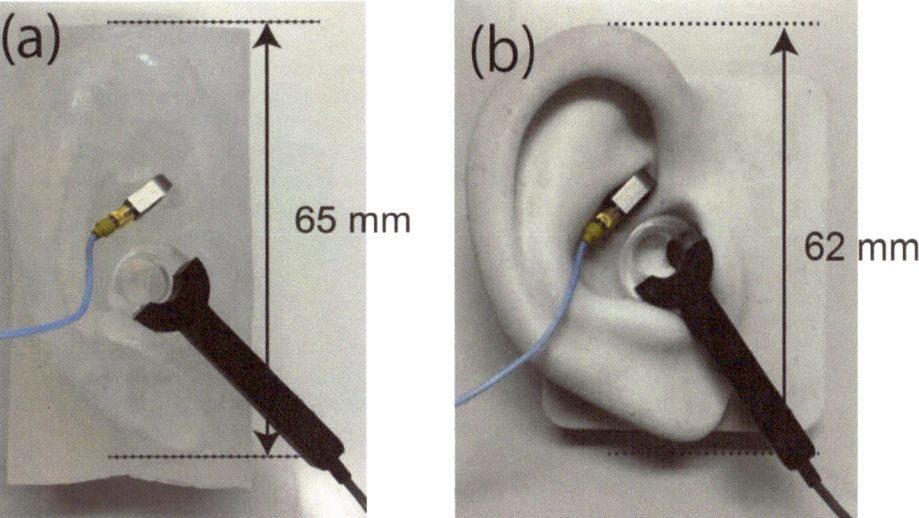

Figure 2. Position of the cartilage conduction transducer and accelerometer of (**a**) pinna simulator made for this study and (**b**) pinna simulator of the HATS.

2. Method

2.1. Pinna Simulators

Various silicon rubbers were molded into the shape of a human pinna and embedded in a base of width × height × thickness: $40 \times 80 \times 40$ mm^3 (Figures 2a and 3). The external auditory canal (inner diameter: 10 mm; length: 35 mm) was excavated within the base. From durometer measurements, the hardness of the various silicon rubbers was classified into five classes: A0, A5, A10, A20, and A40. In addition to these pinna simulators, that of the HATS, with corresponding hardness A5, was used as a reference (Figure 2b).

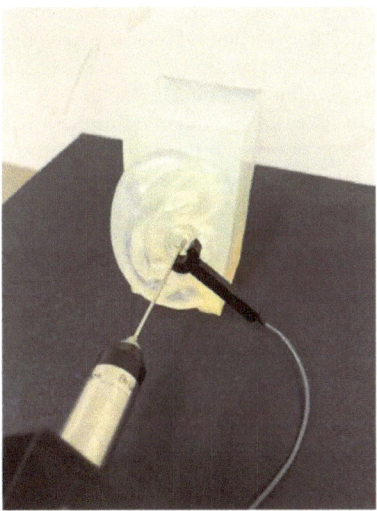

Figure 3. Position of the cartilage conduction transducer and probe microphone of pinna simulator.

2.2. Cartilage Conduction Transducer

In simulations, an annular transducer was used to induce cartilage conduction as in previous measurements [3,6–8,16] (see Figures 2 and 3). The part worn is an acrylic ring (external diameter: 16 mm; internal diameter: 8 mm). The hole acts as an air vent to cancel effects from occlusions and enables cartilage conduction sound in the air canal to be recorded unmodified. The transducer is composed of a piezoelectric bimorph covered with elastic material. Although some resonance peaks appear in the vibrational output, the spectral characteristics are, on the whole, flat in the frequency range above 1 kHz [6]. The cartilage conduction transducer was fixed at the entrance of the external auditory canal between the concha wall and tragus (Figure 2).

2.3. Measurement Procedures for Vibration

The input signal for the transducer is a pure-tone train of frequency ranging from 125 Hz to 16 kHz in 1/12-octave steps. The tones were 1 s in duration, each followed by a silent interval of 0.5 s. The input level was 2.0 V. Vibration acceleration levels (VALs) were determined from the spectral peaks at the corresponding frequencies of the pure tones.

The propagating vibration of the pinna was measured using a subminiature piezotronics accelerometer (model 352A21; PCB Piezotronics, Depew, NY, USA) located on the cymba conchae without any adhesive bond (Figure 2) because a previous study reported that the spectral characteristics of the propagating vibration from the human pinna were not so different among conchae, tragus, and scaphoid fossa, especially below 1 kHz [3]. In addition to the five pinna simulators, the propagating vibration on a human ear (right ear of a male, 42 years old) was measured again for comparison of settings. The hardness of the aural cartilage at the tragus, obtained using a durometer (GS-719N; Teclock, Nagano, Japan), corresponded to A20 or A10. The measured signals were digitized for subsequent analysis with a sampling rate of 44.1 kHz and a 16-bit resolution (UA-101 analog-to-digital converter; Roland, Hamamatsu, Japan).

2.4. Measurement Procedure for Sound

Compared with the vibrational measurement, the procedure used to measure sound in the external auditory canal differed only in the signal receiver. The sound in the auditory canal of the pinna simulator was recorded using a calibrated probe microphone (type 4182; Brüel & Kjaer, Naerum, Denmark), which has a metallic probe tube (length: 100 mm, diameter: 1.24 mm) that allowed sound pressure to be measured in a narrow or enclosed space (Figure 3). The probe was inserted into the external auditory canal through the hole in the annular transducer, without touching it. The tip of the probe was extended 15 mm from the entrance of the auditory canal. The measurement position and procedures were the same as those reported in our previous study [16]. The sound recordings were performed in a soundproof chamber whose background noise was less than 30 dB. Sound pressure levels (SPLs) were determined from the spectral peak at each corresponding frequency of the pure tones.

The SPLs in the auditory canal for the HATS and human ears were extracted from our previous study [16], in which the same cartilage conduction transducer was used. While wearing the transducer (Figure 2b), the SPLs of the HATS were measured as sound passed through the artificial ear mounted on the HATS. The SPLs obtained from the auditory canal of seven participants (25–36 years old) were measured with the same probe microphone (Figure 3) [16]. The SPLs for both the HATS and human ears were comparable to those from current pinna simulators. Before digitizing, the sound output was calibrated using a conditioning amplifier (NEXUS; Brüel & Kjaer, Naerum, Denmark).

3. Results

The VALs obtained from the different pinna simulators were compared with those of a human ear (Figure 4) over the same range of frequencies (<16 kHz). Each curve was determined from the average outputs from three measurements while wearing the accelerometer and transducer and on their removal. Although each line was uneven with small peaks and dips, it was smoothened if the measurement times increased. The standard deviation for each frequency was on average 4.8 dB for A40, 4.9 dB for A20, 5.3 dB for A10, 4.5 dB for A5, 6.1 dB for A0, 3.0 dB for HATS, and 4.9 dB for a human ear.

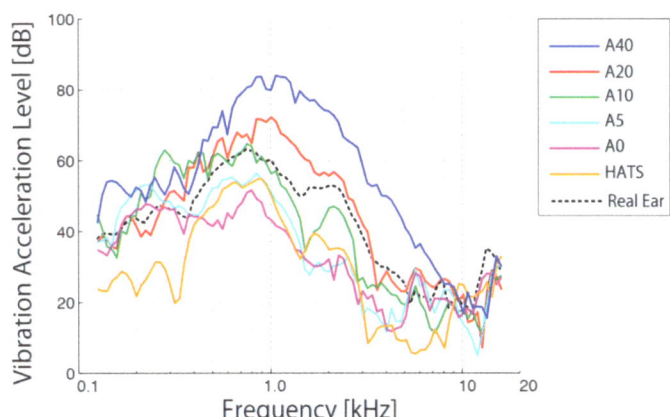

Figure 4. Vibration acceleration level (VAL) as a function of frequency for the various pinna simulators (A40, A20, A10, A5, A0, HATS) and human ear.

The spectral profiles showed a flat or upward trend, up to approximately 1 kHz, and typically decreased after reaching the edge frequency. The characteristics of the peak maxima were 84.0 dB (1059 Hz) for A40, 72.2 dB (1000 Hz) for A 20, 64.8 dB (749 Hz) for A10, 56.5 dB (841 Hz) for A5, 51.7 dB (793 Hz) for A0, 55.0 dB (793 Hz) for HATS, and 63.3 dB (749 Hz) for the human ear. Both peak values and corresponding frequencies decreased with the softening of the pinna hardness. The errors from the VALs of the human ear on average were 14.0 dB for A40, 5.3 dB for A20, 6.4 dB for A10, 9.0 dB for A5, 9.7 dB for A0, and 13.0 dB for HATS.

As for the VAL measurements, the SPLs of the different pinna simulators were measured (Figure 5), each curve being determined from the average outputs among three measurements, while wearing the probe microphone and transducer and on their removal, to assess reproducibility. The standard deviations for each frequency were on average 3.1 dB for A40, 4.7 dB for A20, 2.2 dB for A10, 3.3 dB for A5, and 2.0 dB for A0. The spectral profiles for the HATS and human ear (orange and dashed curves, respectively) are from our previous study [16], in which all measurement instruments and procedures were the same. The value at each frequency was also the average of three measurements obtained from the HATS and the auditory canal of the seven participants.

From the SPLs of the human ear (dashed curve), two clear spectral peaks were evident. The sharp peak at 2.5 kHz arose as a resonance occurring in the external auditory canal, whereas the broad peak at 800 Hz corresponded to sound generated from cartilage conduction [13]. The lower peak disappeared when the transducer was 7 mm distant from the aural cartilage (non-touching condition) [6]. The resonance peak at 2.5 kHz did not change for any of the five pinna simulators because the length of each auditory canal remained the same. However, the peaks arising from cartilage conduction from 700 Hz to 1.5 kHz moved to lower frequencies with the softening of the pinna hardness. The peaks were 90.8 dB (1414 Hz) for A40, 87.2 dB (1000 Hz) for A20, 78.1 dB (561 Hz) for A10, 71.2 dB (944 Hz) for A5, 73.2 dB (891 Hz) for A0, and 75.2 dB (794 Hz) for HATS. As for the vibrational characteristics, both the peak values and corresponding frequencies exhibited a decreasing trend with softening hardness. For the low-frequency range below 1.5 kHz, the errors from the SPLs of the human ear on average were 9.4 dB for A40, 8.3 dB for A20, 4.6 dB for A10, 4.1 dB for A5, 3.7 dB for A0, and 5.7 dB for HATS.

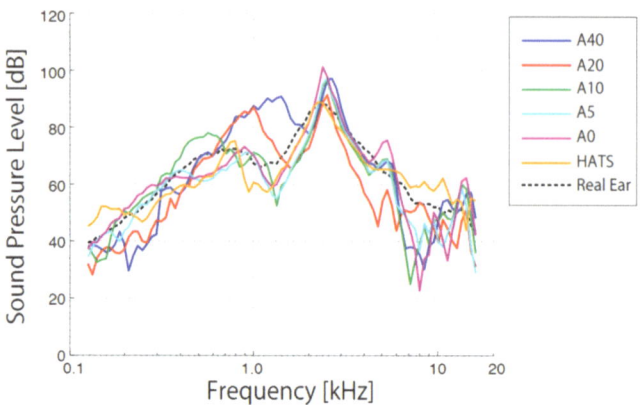

Figure 5. Sound pressure level (SPL) as a function of frequency for the various pinna simulators (A40, A20, A10, A5, A0, HATS) and human ear.

4. Discussion

Silicon rubber has a resonance frequency that depends on Young's modulus (i.e., hardness). One procedure for the measurement of Young's modulus is the dynamical resonance method, which determines Young's modulus (E N/m^2) by measuring the resonance frequency (f Hz) using

$$E = 0.9467 \times \left(\frac{l}{h}\right)^3 \times \frac{m}{w} \times f^2 \quad (1)$$

here, the test sample has mass (m kg) and dimensions (length: (l m), width: (w m), height (h m)) [17]. Although this method applies to steel slabs, Young's modulus of soft silicon rubber is difficult to quantify precisely [18], the resonance frequency being dependent on Young's modulus and hardness.

In the same way, the maximum peaks of propagating vibrations through softer silicon-based pinna simulators were obtained at lower frequencies (Figure 4). Because the pinna simulator of the HATS has a similar hardness of A5, their spectral profiles (cyan and orange curves) are similar. The spectral profiles of the pinna simulators with A20 and A10 (red and green curves) also approximate that of a human ear (black, dashed curve); the averaged VAL errors were lowest for the human ear with hardness A20 and A10. From the hardness measurements obtained using the same durometer, the hardness of the human ear at the tragus corresponded to A20 or A10. These results suggest that vibration simulations of the aural cartilage are important when adjusting the hardness of human aural cartilage. The pinna simulator of the HATS was too soft compared with that for human cartilage and, therefore, in the lower-frequency range below 1.5 kHz. The measured SPLs obtained from the HATS did not agree with those from participants [16].

The results from vibration simulations reflected well the SPL values from the external auditory canal of the pinna simulators (Figure 5). The resonance peaks in cartilage conduction typically appear below 1.5 kHz and move to lower frequencies with the softening of the pinna hardness, similar to the peaks of the VAL curves. The frequencies of the peaks in the SPL curves correlated strongly with those of the VAL curves ($r = 0.89$, $p < 0.01$). When the external auditory canals of participants lying on their sides were filled with water, the hearing threshold of the cartilage conduction lowered at the instant when the water surface reached the aural cartilage [8]. This psycho-acoustical experiment indicated a transmission mechanism in which the vibrating cartilage generates sound in the external auditory canal. Previous physical measurements indicated that certain transducer positions vibrate the aural cartilage more effectively, making sound louder in the external auditory canal [19]. In physical measurements, the VALs in the cartilage and the SPLs in the canal were measured using several transducer positions in the canal entrance of participants, whereas the pinna simulators employed in this study showed a clearer relationship between VAL and SPL because the transducer and accelerometer positions were fixed.

In the lower-frequency range below 1.5 kHz, the peak frequency of the SPL for the human ear (749 Hz) was between that for A20 (1000 Hz) and A10 (561 Hz). Similar to the vibration results, the results agreed with the hardness of actual aural cartilage subjected to sound pressures of a similar spectral profile. While the hardness set for the pinna simulators for the HATS was too soft to simulate the vibration in a human aural cartilage, the artificial ear embedded in the HATS could precisely simulate the behavior in the higher-frequency range above 1.5 kHz [16]. In a future study, pinna simulators of differing hardness for the HATS are to be made, and the sound output will be compared with the measured SPLs from the ears of participants. Following the conclusions obtained from the abovementioned results, the simulated SPL is expected to agree with the measured data when the hardness of the pinna simulator approximates that of human aural cartilage.

Limitation of the Study

In this study, the hardness of aural cartilage was measured by one participant (male, 42 years old) whose pinna did not have any disorder. However, it is possible that the hardness of aural cartilage may be varied according to the age, sex, and disorder, and the vibrational and acoustical characteristics of the cartilage conduction may be changed as the results. Further study is required to examine statistical analyses regarding the hardness.

5. Conclusions

Using five pinna simulators differing in hardness, vibrations at the pinna and sound in the external auditory canal were measured and compared with those of a human ear for the purpose of calibrating cartilage conduction of sound. From VAL and SPL curves, we found that the spectral characteristics for the pinna simulators approached those of the human ears when their hardness coincided. The simulation of cartilage conduction of sound using the HATS is possible if the hardness of the pinna simulator is adjusted to that of human aural cartilage.

Author Contributions: The conceptualization, methodology, data analysis, and original draft preparation of this study were developed by R.S. and the discussion and subsequent conclusion were supervised by H.H. and T.N. All authors have read and agreed to the published version of the manuscript.

Funding: This research was supported by a Grant-in-Aid for Science Research (B) from the Japan Society for the Promotion of Science (18H03560).

Institutional Review Board Statement: Ethical review and approval were waived for this study, because wearing cartilage conduction transducer, whose output is limited below 1 V, does not have any risk for hearing loss.

Informed Consent Statement: Informed consent was obtained from all subjects involved in the study.

Data Availability Statement: Not applicable.

Acknowledgments: The authors thank the participants for their cooperation during the experiment. In addition, we thank Takashi Iwakura and Kyoji Yoshikawa (Rion Co., Ltd.) for prototyping the cartilage-conduction hearing aids. Additionally, we thank R.W. Haase for editing a draft of this manuscript.

Conflicts of Interest: The authors declare no conflict of interest.

References

1. Hosoi, H. Receiver. Japanese Patent Application Number 166644, 4 June 2004.
2. Hosoi, H. Approach in the Use of Cartilage Conduction Speaker. Japanese Patent Number 4541111, 17 November 2004.
3. Shimokura, R.; Hosoi, H.; Iwakura, T.; Nishimura, T.; Matsui, T. Development of monaural and binaural behind-the-ear cartilage conduction hearing aids. *Appl. Acoust.* **2013**, *74*, 1234–1240. [CrossRef]
4. Nishimura, T.; Hosoi, H.; Sugiuchi, T.; Matsumoto, N.; Nishiyama, T.; Takano, K.; Sugimoto, S.; Yazama, H.; Sato, T.; Komori, M. Cartilage conduction hearing aid fitting in clinical practice. *J. Am. Acad. Audiol.* **2021**. [CrossRef]

5. Nishimura, T.; Hosoi, H.; Shimokura, R.; Morimoto, C.; Kitahara, T. Cartilage conduction hearing and its clinical application. *Audiol. Res.* **2021**, *11*, 254–262. [CrossRef]
6. Shimokura, R.; Hosoi, H.; Nishimura, T.; Yamanaka, T.; Levitt, H. Cartilage conduction hearing. *J. Acoust. Soc. Am.* **2014**, *135*, 1959–1966. [CrossRef] [PubMed]
7. Nishimura, T.; Hosoi, H.; Saito, O.; Miyamae, R.; Shimokura, R.; Matsui, T.; Yamanaka, T.; Levitt, H. Is cartilage conduction classified into air or bone conduction? *Laryngoscope* **2014**, *124*, 1214–1219. [CrossRef] [PubMed]
8. Nishimura, T.; Hosoi, H.; Saito, O.; Miyamae, R.; Shimokura, R.; Yamanaka, T.; Kitahara, T.; Levitt, H. Cartilage conduction is characterized by vibrations of the cartilaginous portion of the ear canal. *PLoS ONE* **2015**, *10*, e0120135. [CrossRef] [PubMed]
9. Hosoi, H.; Nishimura, T.; Shimokura, R.; Kitahara, T. Cartilage conduction as the third pathway for sound transmission. *Auris Nasus Larynx* **2019**, *46*, 151–159. [CrossRef] [PubMed]
10. Morimoto, C.; Nishimura, T.; Hosoi, H.; Saito, O.; Fukuda, F.; Shimokura, R.; Yamanaka, T. Sound transmission of cartilage conduction in the ear with fibrotic aural atresia. *J. Rehabil. Res. Dev.* **2014**, *51*, 325–332. [CrossRef] [PubMed]
11. Nishimura, T.; Hosoi, H.; Saito, O.; Shimokura, R.; Yamanaka, T.; Kitahara, T. Cartilage conduction hearing aids for sever conduction hearing loss. *Otol. Neurotol.* **2018**, *39*, 65–72. [CrossRef] [PubMed]
12. ISO 389-2, *Acoustics—Reference zero for the Calibration of Audiometric Equipment—Part 2: Reference Equivalent Threshold Sound Pressure Levels for Pure Tones and Insert Earphones*; International Organization for Standardization: Geneva, Switzerland, 1994.
13. ISO 389-3, *Acoustics—Reference Zero for the Calibration of Audiometric Equipment—Part 3: Reference Equivalent Threshold Force Levels for Pure Tones and Bone Vibrators*; International Organization for Standardization: Geneva, Switzerland, 1994.
14. IEC 60318-7, *Electroacoustics—Simulations of Human Head and Ear—Part 7: Head and Torso Simulator for the Measurement of Hearing Aids*; International Electrotechnical Commission: Geneva, Switzerland, 2011.
15. IEC 60318-4, *Electroacoustics—Simulations of Human Head and Ear—Part 4: Occluded-Ear Simulator for the Measurement of Earphones Coupled to the Ear by Means of Ear Inserts*; International Electrotechnical Commission: Geneva, Switzerland, 2010.
16. Shimokura, R.; Hosoi, H.; Nishimura, T.; Iwakura, T.; Yamanaka, T. Simulating cartilage conduction sound to estimate the sound pressure level in the external auditory canal. *J. Sound Vib.* **2015**, *335*, 261–268. [CrossRef]
17. JIS Z 2280-1993, *Test Method for Young's Modulus of Metallic Materials at Elevated Temperature*; Japanese Industrial Standards Committee: Tokyo, Japan, 1993.
18. Gent, A.N. On the relation between indentation hardness and Young's modulus. *Inst. Rubber Ind. Trans.* **1958**, *34*, 46–57. [CrossRef]
19. Pampush, J.D.; Daegling, D.J.; Vick, A.E.; Mcgraw, W.S.; Covey, R.M.; Rapoff, A. Technical Note: Converting durometer data into elastic modulus in biological materials. *Am. J. Phys. Anthropol.* **2011**, *146*, 650–653. [CrossRef] [PubMed]

Article
Clinical Trial for Cartilage Conduction Hearing Aid in Indonesia

Ronny Suwento [1,*], Dini Widiarni Widodo [1,*], Tri Juda Airlangga [1], Widayat Alviandi [1], Keisuke Watanuki [2], Naoko Nakanowatari [2], Hiroshi Hosoi [3] and Tadashi Nishimura [3]

1. Department of Otorhinolaryngology Head and Neck Surgery, Cipto Mangunkusumo Hospital—Faculty of Medicine, Universitas Indonesia, Jakarta 10430, Indonesia; airlanggamd@gmail.com (T.J.A.); widayat_alviandi@yahoo.com (W.A.)
2. RION Co., Tokyo 185-8533, Japan; watanuki@rion.co.jp (K.W.); naoko@rion.co.jp (N.N.)
3. Nara Medical University, Kashihara 634-8522, Nara, Japan; hosoi@naramed-u.ac.jp (H.H.); t-nishim@naramed-u.ac.jp (T.N.)
* Correspondence: rsuwanto@yahoo.com (R.S.); dini_pancho@yahoo.com (D.W.W.)

Abstract: Hearing improvement represents one of the may valuable outcomes in microtia and aural atresia reconstruction surgery. Most patients with poor development in their hearing function have had a severe microtia. Conventional methods to improve hearing function are bone conduction and bone anchored hearing aids. Cartilage conduction hearing aids (CCHA) represents a new amplification method. This study assessed the outcomes and evaluated the impact and its safety in the patients with microtia and aural atresia whose hearing dysfunction did not improve after surgery for ear reconstruction in our hospital. Hearing functions were evaluated with pure tone audiometry or sound field testing by behavioral audiometry and speech audiometry before and after CCHA fitting. As a result, there was a significant difference between unaided and aided thresholds ($p < 0.001$). Speech recognition threshold and speech discrimination level also significantly improved with CCHA. The average functional gains of 14 ears were 26.9 ± 2.3 dB. Almost all parents of the patients reported satisfaction with the performance of CCHA, and daily communication in children with hearing loss also became better than usual.

Keywords: cartilage conduction hearing aid; microtia; hearing function; clinical trial

1. Introduction

Microtia is a congenital auricular malformation that usually occurs in conjunction with ear canal atresia, and ranges from mild structural abnormalities to the complete absence of the ear (anotia). It can occur unilaterally or bilaterally. In unilateral cases, the right side is more affected. The prevalence rate of microtia ranges from 0.83 to 17.4 per 10,000 [1]. In the ENT outpatient clinic, Dr. Cipto Mangunkusumo National Hospital, Jakarta, there were 207 microtia ears in 2008–2014, and 173 ears underwent surgery in the patients aged from 6 to 12 years of age. Between 2017 and 2018, there were 32 new microtia cases, aged between 1 month and 14 years. Male babies have been more frequently affected than female babies (2:1).

Microtia patients have three main problems, namely functional, aesthetic, and psychosocial problems [1]. Microtia surgery has been proved to lower psychological stressors which may impact the mental development of children with microtia [2]. Hearing habilitation for infants and children with microtia who are still in developing age should be performed without waiting for reconstructive surgery. One of the options for microtia hearing habilitation that is commonly used in Indonesia is the installation of bone conduction hearing aid. However, this method is ineffective due to several obstacles such as the difficulty in obtaining the correct hearing aid input, transducer pressure (which makes it unstable on bones), the occurrence of skin laceration due to transducer pressure, and its higher cost than air conductive hearing aids. Another option is the installation of a bone anchored hearing aid (BAHA), which is even more expensive and requires surgery. In addition, complications can also occur after the BAHA implantation surgery [3–5].

When children become old enough to undergo ear reconstruction surgery, hearing habilitation can be assisted by performing atresiaplasty. Hearing improvement becomes one of valuable outcomes of microtia reconstruction surgery [2]. About 64% patients gain significant hearing improvement after atresiaplasty. This result remained stable for up to three years post-surgery. Most patients who did not develop their hearing function had a severe degree of microtia. Severe malformed middle ear and stenosis of the ear canal are associated with a negative impact on auditory development [2,6]. However, atresiaplasty is also often a dilemma since it can result in restenosis of the ear canal. Ear canal restenosis is caused by circumference wounds (360°) that can cause contractures as well as fibrosis of the soft tissue around the wound. These factors cause the amplification effort to be hampered so that the patient still has hearing problems after the reconstruction procedure [7].

Hearing amplification technology development is needed to overcome these obstacles, especially for infants and children. Cartilage conduction hearing aid (CCHA) developed by Hosoi and colleagues provides new hope and can be an alternative option for overcoming hearing amplification problems in microtia cases [8–12]. Cartilage conduction is a newly suggested transduction form whose characteristics are different from air and bone conductions. [13–20] CCHA has several advantages such as sound clarity, sound localization, and more stable connection between the transducer and the cartilage surface [20–22]. The transducer can be attached to the cartilage part in humans via a special double-sided tape. As previous studies stated [12,23–27], CCHA can be used for sound transmission even in aural atresia. Most issues with bone conduction (BC) hearing aids are related to the properties of the transducer and the form of conduction. For cartilage conduction (CC), the transducer is designed to vibrate the aural cartilage rather than the skull bone; therefore, it is small and lightweight. By inserting the transducer into the cavity of the concha, a headband is not needed for fixation. It is held in place by the combination of its own weight and the stiffness of the concha cartilage. In addition to its cosmetic advantages, the fixation of a CC transducer is more comfortable and convenient than that of a BC transducer [12]. This alternative conduction method may solve the issues related to BC hearing aids.

The purpose of this clinical trial is to find out whether CCHA is useful for patients with severe conductive hearing loss due to aural atresia. This study also aimed to assess the outcomes and to evaluate the impact and safety of CCHA in the patients with microtia and aural atresia whose hearing dysfunction were difficult to improve by following ear surgery reconstruction at the ENT Department, Dr. Cipto Mangunkusumo National Hospital, Jakarta.

2. Method

2.1. Participants

This is a quasi-experimental study comparing outcomes before and after intervention. We used purposive sampling to choose subjects based on inclusion criteria. This clinical trial was conducted at the ENT Department, Dr Cipto Mangunkusumo National Hospital—Faculty of Medicine Universitas Indonesia, Jakarta from August 2019 to January 2020. This study has been approved by the Ethics Committee of Faculty of Medicine, Universitas Indonesia with an official letter of 17 June 2019, Number KET/UN2/ETIK/PPM.00.02/2019 with Protocol number: 19-05-0533. We clarify cases which were suitable to our inclusion criteria. Subjects with sensorineural hearing loss were excluded. Subjects' parents were provided written informed consent after being informed the nature of the procedure and purpose of this study.

The present study evaluated 10 children diagnosed as microtia and aural atresia. Six subjects (60%) were female and four were males (40%). Eight subjects had bilateral microtia and aural atresia while the other two subjects were only one ear (unilateral). The total number involved 18 ears (8 right ears and 10 left ears) of microtia and aural atresia.

Subjects' average age was 12.4 ± 3.1 years; the youngest was 9 years while the oldest was 19 years. All subjects were classified as microtia grade III, with a Jahrsdoerfer score less than 7. All subjects had undergone auricular and aural atresia reconstruction surgery and did not get hearing improvement after surgery. Only one patient (number 10) had ever used conventional bone conduction hearing aid bilaterally, but it had been used for only four months because of discomfort. In patient nine, Bone anchored hearing aid (BAHA) was installed before but was released due to complications (excessive granulation tissue).

Initially, we filled in the complete identity of the subjects in the research form, interviewed the parents, and reviewed the subjects' medical records. This was followed by air and bone conduction pure tone audiometry or behavioral audiometry or bone conduction ABR, and speech audiometry. Clinical audiometer (AC 40; Interacoustics, Middelfart, Denmark) and ABR Bio-Logic Navigator Pro (Natus Medical Inc., San Carlos, CA, USA) were used for the measurement. Speech audiometry was performed using Otometrics Madsen Astera (Natus, Taastrup, Denmark). In the initial audiology test, only seven patients completed pure tone audiometry, with average hearing threshold taken from 500, 1000, 2000 and 4000 Hz. The other three patients were not cooperative to have pure tone audiometry performed; subjective auditory responses were evaluated with behavioral audiometry in one of them and the audiology response of the other two patients were determined based on the tone burst (TB) bone conduction ABR.

Based on the results of the initial audiological tests, the diagnosis of hearing loss in 18 ears was conductive hearing loss with a degree of profound hearing loss in 2 ears, severe hearing loss in 12 ears, and 4 moderate hearing loss (Table 1).

Table 1. Characteristics of 10 Patients with Microtia and Aural Atresia.

Patient	Sex	Age (Year)	Pure Tone/Behavioral Audiometry (dB HL) [500, 1000, 2000, 4000 Hz]		TB Bone ABR (dB nHL)		Degree of Conductive Hearing Loss	
			R	L	R	L	R	L
1	F	13	107.5/67.5	101.3/68.8	-	-	Profound/Severe	Profound/Severe
2	M	9	NA/50	NA/50	-	-	-/Moderate	-/Moderate
3	F	14	66.3/62.5	62.5/53.8	-	-	Severe/Severe	Severe/Moderate
4	F	10	NA	NA	60	60	Severe	Severe
5	M	9	NA	NA	55	65	Moderate	Severe
6	M	12	60.0/51.3	61.3/56.3	-	-	Severe/Moderate	Severe/Moderate
7	F	13	70.0/32.5	58.8/28.8	-	-	Severe/Mild	Moderate/Mild
8	F	19	Normal/Normal	68.8/70.0	-	-	Normal/Normal	Severe/Severe
9	F	15	Normal/Normal	82.5/82.5	-	-	Normal/Normal	Severe/Severe
10	F	10	61.3/68.8	65.0/65.0	-	-	Severe/Severe	Severe/Severe

M, male; F, female; R, right ear; L, left ear; NA, not available; ABR, auditory brainstem response.

2.2. CCHA Fitting and Evaluations

HB-J1CC CCHA (Rion Co. Ltd., Tokyo, Japan) was used for CCHA fitting (Figure 1a). An ear impression was taken to prepare the CCHA transducer when the ear-chip type transducer was necessary. CCHAs with ear-chip type transducer were fitted in patient three (left ear) and five (both ears), while the simple type transducer was affixed to the external ear cartilage with a double-sided skin tape (#1522; 3M Japan Limited, Tokyo, Japan) in others (Figure 1b). The transducers were placed on the tragal area which consist mostly of cartilage. CCHA adjustments was performed based on functional gains. Unaided and aided thresholds were measured in the same day by sound field test, and functional gains were obtained.

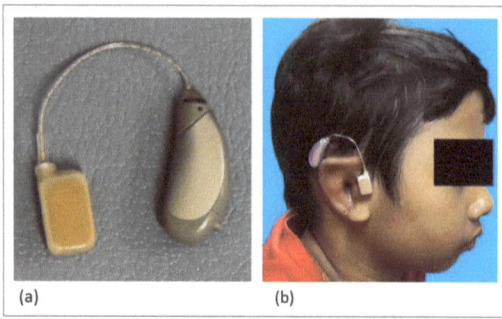

Figure 1. Cartilage conduction hearing aid (**a**) and the appearance of it on a patient ear (**b**).

Speech audiometry assessments were also performed by calculating speech recognition threshold (SRT) and speech discrimination score (SDS). The intensity level at which the patient could correctly repeat 50% of spondee words (single words which comprise two syllables with equal emphasis placed on each syllable) was measured and defined as SRT. The SRTs should correspond roughly to the average pure tone audiometry thresholds at 500, 1000 and 2000 Hz. Meanwhile, The SDS (also called word recognition score) is a score of the number of words correctly repeated, expressed as a percentage of correct (discrimination score) or incorrect (discrimination loss).

Furthermore, speech discrimination level (SDL) was defined as the lowest level at which enough SDS was obtained for communication. SDL indicates the patient's ability to hear and understand speech at typical conversation levels, which helps us to predict the potential benefits from the amplification.

The final session incorporated with sound field testing (unaided and aided) and the subjective benefits of CCHA use in a daily life were evaluated with a questionnaire for parents.

3. Results

Hearing threshold improvements which are assessed based on functional gain were performed in 14 ears. The functional gains were obtained as the result of the difference value between aided and unaided audiometric behavioral threshold. Patient one, four, and five were difficult to perform hearing and speech examination and CCHA fitting on. It should be explained that the results of behavioral audiometry in patient one are inconsistent during the three months of the examination sessions. The patient's emotions during examination sessions were unstable. The same condition also happened to patients four and five, who were not cooperative. However, at the last session, the behavioral audiometry was successfully conducted in patient four, as the results were reliable. Patient five could not produce any reliable result because of their uncooperativeness. Thus, we fitted their CCHA based on their previous bone conduction ABR result. Nonetheless, patients one, four, and five were subjectively seen more comfortable and wanted to wear CCHA.

Functional gains could be obtained in 14 ears of 8 patients. Obtained values ranged from 11.25 dB to 46.25 dB (Table 2). The average functional gain of 14 ears was 26.9 ± 2.3 dB. The greatest improvements in hearing threshold among the bilateral fitting cases were 35 and 38.75 dB in patient four. For unilateral fitting cases, the largest functional gain was 46.25 dB observed in the left ear of patient nine.

Table 2. CCHA fitting and its outcome.

Patient	Ear-Chip	DFT	Ear	Unaided/Aided Thresholds (dB HL)	Functional Gain (dB)	Unaided/Aided SRTs (dB HL)	SRT-I (dB)	Unaided/Aided SDLs (dB HL)	SDL-I (dB)
1	No	Yes	R	NC/90	NC	NC	NC	NC	NC
	No	Yes	L	NC/68.8	NC	NC	NC	NC	NC
2	No	Yes	R	50/27.5	22.5	68/46	22	100/60	40
	No	Yes	L	50.0/28.8	21.3	72/47	25	100/60	40
3	No	Yes	R	52.5/31.3	21.3	93/49	44	NC/90	-
	Yes	No	L	48.8/37.5	11.3	82/60	22	100/80	20
4	No	Yes	R	66.3/31.3	35.0	NC	NC	NC	NC
	No	Yes	L	63.8/25.0	38.8	NC	NC	NC	NC
5	Yes	No	R	NC	NC	NC	NC	NC	NC
	Yes	No	L	NC	NC	NC	NC	NC	NC
6	No	Yes	R	50.0/27,5	22.5	75/30	45	?/60	-
	No	Yes	L	50.0/28.8	21.3	92/28	64	100/60	40
7	No	Yes	R	65.0/38.8	26.3	81/42	39	90/50	40
	No	Yes	L	56.3/30.0	26.3	73/37	36	80/50	30
8	-	-	R	Normal	-	-	-	-	-
	No	Yes	L	68.8/38.8	30.0	74/50	24	90/60	30
9	-	-	R	Normal	-	-	-	-	-
	No	Yes	L	76.3/30.0	46.3	85/50	35	90/60	30
10	No	Yes	R	57.5/32.5	25.0	76/28	48	90/50	40
	No	Yes	L	61.3/32.5	28.8	75/42	33	90/50	40

DFT: double-sided tape for transducer and hearing aid unit; SRT: speech recognition score; SDL: speech discrimination level; I: improvement; R: Right ear; L: Left ear; NC: not cooperative.

A statistical test was performed to evaluate the outcome significance. Firstly, a Shapiro–Wilk test was conducted to evaluate data normality for subjects with less than 50 samples. As the P value is higher than 0.05, data distribution was normal and mean and standard deviation were used to present the data. Secondly, parametric statistical test was performed. Based on the paired T-test, mean difference of functional gain obtained was 26.9 ± 2.3 dB (95% CI). It was concluded that there is a statistically significant difference ($p < 0.001$) in the average hearing threshold between unaided and aided conditions. (Table 3).

Table 3. Averaged unaided/aided thresholds and functional gain.

Unaided Threshold (n = 14)	Aided Threshold (n = 14)	Functional Gain (95% Confidence Interval)	P Value (Paired T-Test)
58.3 ± 2.3 dB HL	31.4 ± 1.1 dB HL	26.9 ± 2.3 dB	<0.001

SRT results were successfully obtained in 12 ears of 7 patients. SRT results was improved in all seven patients, with improvements ranged from 24 to 64 dB (Table 2). The average SRT improvement was 36.4 ± 12.6 dB. Improvement of SDL values also occurred in all seven subjects with median value of 40 dB and minimum and maximal values of 20 dB and 40 dB, respectively (Table 2). The smallest aided SDL value recorded was 50 dB. The SDL improvement in patients with CCHA might be larger than the obtained values.

Almost all subjects' parents reported satisfaction with the performance of CCHA; subject daily communication becomes better, and it was reported that the subjects felt more comfortable with CCHA installed. After six months of CCHA installation, no disturbing problems have been reported. No adverse effects or allergies were found due to double-sided tape. The results of the evaluation of hearing aid adaptability test questionnaire to subjects' parents were as follows: good adaptability (90%); the effect of improvement was felt immediately (85%); ease operability factor (90%); device appearance (100%); and comfort of use (90%).

4. Discussions

Overall, the hearing threshold (functional gain), and the ability to understand speech (speech audiometry) of all subjects improved after CCHA installation, which agreed with the previous clinical trial [12]. The benefit obtained by CCHA users in this study were not the same but varied. This variable benefit might result from the individual pathology. A person might have poorer speech discrimination scores than others due to the way the cochlear hair cells or auditory nerve had been damaged. It might also be due to a patient's personality, or a combination of other factors.

One of the difficulties in determining the audiological status of a patient with microtia and aural atresia is a psychosocial problem that causes difficulties in performing a hearing examination. This has been conveyed in various studies including by Li et.al., who studied 170 microtia patients [28]. They reported that microtia and aural atresia patients aged 8–10 years (boy) and 11–13 years (girl) had a high incidence of social problems in the form of interpersonal sensitivity, depression, anxiety, and hostility. This also occurred in the microtia and aural atresia patients in our study, which consisted of 6 girls and 4 boys, with an age range of 9–19 years, so that only 6 patients could undergo pure tone audiometry. As an alternative procedure, behavioral audiometry was performed for 8 patients (12 ears), while 2 other patients, aged 10 and 9 years, were still unable to undergo behavioral audiometry. In these two patients, bone conduction ABR, allowing the identification of the type and the degree of conduction hearing loss, was performed to assess the cochlear integrity [29]. Due to psychosocial problems, the two subjects could not complete another audiological test session. However, the parents of both subjects still wanted to participate in the installation of the CCHA, and both subjects felt better subjectively after using CCHA.

Evaluating the performance in the patients with difficulty in behavioral audiometry, the real ear measurement is effective in normal anatomical ears [30], and the simulator for CC is also beneficial to the estimation [31,32]. Unfortunately, the ear canal was substantially absent in the atretic ears, and these measurements cannot exactly reflect the signal transmission to the cochlea. Technological developments in objectively evaluating the performance in the atretic ears are necessary since a suitable candidate for CCHA is a patient with aural atresia. Subject parents reported that the CCHA unit was very light, relatively small in size, and that it therefore looks better cosmetically. Most of the subjects used double-sided tape for fixation of transducers and hearing aid units; only two subjects could use the ear-chip type transducer. Sound transmission is quite good with the use of double-sided tape and does not cause pressure on the skin attachment. The similar audiometric outcomes have been reported by Nishimura et al. [12]. The style of the transducer fixation using double-sided tapes and the type of aural atresia had no significant influence on the functional gains [12].

The limitation of this study is its small sample size as we only had 10 subjects who met the inclusion criteria. In addition, the subject was difficult to follow up due to the travel restriction policy during Covid-19 pandemic. Some of them also had psychosocial problem that cause difficulties in performing hearing tests.

5. Conclusions

The CCHA outcome and benefits in this study were varied. This is caused by different respond to the device. This variable benefit may also result from individual pathology. Based on audiometric tests and interviews with the subject parents, CCHA is a hearing aid choice that provides optimal hearing amplification. CCHA is a suitable and profitable option of hearing rehabilitation for microtia and aural atresia patients who do not receive benefit or amplification following ear reconstruction surgery.

Author Contributions: Conceptualization, R.S., D.W.W., T.N. and H.H.; methodology, D.W.W.; software, T.J.A., W.A.; validation, R.S.; formal analysis, R.S., D.W.W. and T.N.; investigation, R.S., D.W.W., K.W., T.J.A. and W.A.; resources, R.S., D.W.W.; data curation, R.S., D.W.W.; statistic analytic, D.W.W.; writing—original draft preparation, R.S., D.W.W.; writing—review and editing, R.S., D.W.W.

and T.N.; visualization, R.S.; supervision, H.H.; project administration, K.W.; funding acquisition, N.N. All authors have read and agreed to the published version of the manuscript.

Funding: This research received 18 Cartilage Conduction Hearing Aid and already install for 10 (ten) microtia patients and funding for journal publication from RION Co, Japan.

Institutional Review Board Statement: The study was conducted according to the guidelines of the Declaration of Helsinki and approved by the Ethics Committee of Faculty of Medicine Universitas Indonesia with an official letter of 17 June 2019 Number KET/UN2/ETIK/PPM.00.02/2019 with Protocol number: 19-05-0533.

Informed Consent Statement: Informed consent was obtained from all subject parents involved in the study.

Data Availability Statement: The data used to support the findings of this study are available within the article.

Conflicts of Interest: The authors declare no conflict of interest.

References

1. Sanjib, T.; Meng, X. Treatment of Microtia: Past, Present and Future. *J. Southeast Univ.* **2015**, *34*, 485–488. [CrossRef]
2. Pellinen, J.; Vasama, J.P.; Kivekäs, I. Long-term Results of Atresiaplasty in Patients with Congenital Aural Atresia. *Acta Oto-Laryngol.* **2018**, *138*, 1–4. [CrossRef]
3. Håkansson, B.; Tjellström, A.; Rosenhall, U. Hearing Thresholds with Direct Bone Conduction Versus Conventional Bone Conduction. *Scand Audiol.* **1984**, *13*, 3–13. [CrossRef] [PubMed]
4. House, J.W.; Kutz, J.W. Bone-anchored Hearing Aids: Incidence and Management of Postoperative Complications. *Otol. Neurotol.* **2007**, *28*, 213–217. [CrossRef] [PubMed]
5. Hobson, J.C.; Roper, A.J.; Andrew, R.; Rothera, M.P.; Hill, P.; Green, K.M. Complications of Bone-anchored Hearing Aid Implantation. *J. Laryngol. Otol.* **2010**, *124*, 132–136. [CrossRef]
6. Chang, S.O.; Choi, B.Y.; Hur, D.G. Analysis of the Long-Term Hearing Results After the Surgical Repair of Aural Atresia. *Laryngoscope* **2006**, *116*, 1835–1841. [CrossRef] [PubMed]
7. Başerer, N. The Experience Outcomes of the Cosmetic and Functional Surgery in Congenital Aural Atresia. *Clin. Surg.* **2017**, *2*, 1–5.
8. Hosoi, H.; Yanai, S.; Nishimura, T.; Sakaguchi, T.; Iwakura, T.; Yoshino, K. Development of cartilage con-duction hearing aid. *Arch. Mat. Sci. Eng.* **2010**, *42*, 104–110.
9. Nishimura, T.; Hosoi, H.; Saito, O.; Miyamae, R.; Shimokura, R.; Matsui, T.; Iwakura, T. Benefit of a New Hearing Device Utilizing Cartilage Conduction. *Auris Nasus Larynx* **2013**, *40*, 440–446. [CrossRef]
10. Shimokura, R.; Hosoi, H.; Iwakura, T.; Nishimura, T.; Matsui, T. Development of monaural and binaural behind-the-ear cartilage conduction hearing aids. *Appl. Acoust.* **2013**, *74*, 1234–1240. [CrossRef]
11. Nishimura, T.; Hosoi, H.; Sugiuchi, T.; Matsumoto, N.; Nishiyama, T.; Takano, K.; Sugimoto, S.; Yazama, H.; Sato, T.; Komori, M. Cartilage conduction hearing aid fitting in clinical practice. *J. Am. Acad. Audiol.* **2021**, in press.
12. Nishimura, T.; Hosoi, H.; Saito, O.; Shimokura, R.; Yamanaka, T.; Kitahara, T. Cartilage Conduction Hearing Aids for Severe Conduction Hearing Loss. *Otol. Neurotol.* **2018**, *39*, 65–72. [CrossRef]
13. Nishimura, T.; Hosoi, H.; Saito, O.; Miyamae, R.; Shimokura, R.; Matsui, T.; Yamanaka, T.; Levitt, H. Is cartilage conduction classified into air or bone conduction? *Laryngoscope.* **2014**, *124*, 1214–1219. [CrossRef] [PubMed]
14. Shimokura, R.; Hosoi, H.; Nishimura, T.; Yamanaka, T.; Levitt, H. Cartilage conduction hearing. *J. Acoust Soc. Am.* **2014**, *135*, 1959–1966. [CrossRef] [PubMed]
15. Nishimura, T.; Hosoi, H.; Saito, O.; Miyamae, R.; Shimokura, R.; Yamanaka, T.; Kitahara, T.; Levitt, H. Cartilage conduction is characterized by vibrations of the cartilaginous portion of the ear canal. *PLoS ONE* **2015**, *10*, e0120135. [CrossRef]
16. Nishimura, T.; Hosoi, H.; Saito, O.; Miyamae, R.; Shimokura, R.; Matsui, T.; Yamanaka, T.; Kitahara, T.; Levitt, H. Cartilage conduction efficiently generates airborne sound in the ear canal. *Auris Nasus Larynx.* **2015**, *42*, 15–19. [CrossRef]
17. Miyamae, R.; Nishimura, T.; Hosoi, H.; Saito, O.; Shimokura, R.; Yamanaka, T.; Kitahara, T. Perception of speech in cartilage conduction. *Auris Nasus Larynx.* **2017**, *44*, 26–32. [CrossRef]
18. Nishimura, T.; Miyamae, R.; Hosoi, H.; Saito, O.; Shimokura, R.; Yamanaka, T.; Kitahara, T. Frequency characteristics and speech recognition in cartilage conduction. *Auris Nasus Larynx.* **2019**, *46*, 709–715. [CrossRef]
19. Nishimura, T.; Hosoi, H.; Saito, O.; Akasaka, S.; Shimokura, R.; Yamanaka, T.; Kitahara, T. Effect of fixation place on airborne sound in cartilage conduction. *J. Acoust. Soc. Am.* **2020**, *148*, 469. [CrossRef]
20. Nishimura, T.; Hosoi, H.; Shimokura, R.; Morimoto, C.; Kitahara, T. Cartilage Conduction Hearing and Its Clinical Application. *Audiol. Res.* **2021**, *11*, 254–262. [CrossRef]
21. Hosoi, H.; Nishimura, T.; Shimokura, R.; Kitahara, T. Cartilage conduction as the third pathway for sound transmission. *Auris Nasus Larynx.* **2019**, *46*, 151–159. [CrossRef]

22. Nishimura, T.; Hosoi, H.; Saito, O.; Shimokura, R.; Yamanaka, T.; Kitahara, T. Sound localisation ability using cartilage conduction hearing aids in bilateral aural atresia. *Int. J. Audiol.* **2020**, *59*, 891–896. [CrossRef]
23. Morimoto, C.; Nishimura, T.; Hosoi, H.; Saito, O.; Fukuda, F.; Shimokura, R.; Yamanaka, T. Sound transmis-sion by cartilage conduction in ear with fibrotic aural atresia. *J. Rehabil. Res. Dev.* **2014**, *51*, 325–332. [CrossRef] [PubMed]
24. Nishiyama, T.; Oishi, N.; Ogawa, K. Who are good adult candidates for cartilage conduction hearing aids? *Eur. Arch. Otorhinolaryngol.* **2020**, in press. [CrossRef] [PubMed]
25. Nishiyama, T.; Oishi, N.; Ogawa, K. Efficacy of cartilage conduction hearing aids in children. *Int. J. Pediatr Otorhinolaryngol.* **2021**, *142*, 110628. [CrossRef]
26. Komune, N.; Higashino, Y.; Ishikawa, K.; Tabuki, T.; Masuda, S.; Koike, K.; Hongo, T.; Sato, K.; Uchi, R.; Miyazaki, M.; et al. Management of Residual Hearing with Cartilage Conduction Hearing Aid after Lateral Temporal Bone Resection: Our Institutional Experience. *Audiol. Res.* **2021**, *11*, 263–274. [CrossRef] [PubMed]
27. Akasaka, S.; Nishimura, T.; Hosoi, H.; Saito, O.; Shimokura, R.; Morimoto, C.; Kitahara, T. Benefits of Cartilage Conduction Hearing Aids for Speech Perception in Unilateral Aural Atresia. *Audiol. Res.* **2021**, *11*, 284–290. [CrossRef] [PubMed]
28. Li, D.; Chin, W.; Wu, J.; Zhang, Q.; Xu, F.; Zhang, R. Psychosocial Outcomes Among Microtia Patients of Different Ages and Genders Before Ear Reconstruction. *Aesthetic Plast. Surg.* **2010**, *34*, 570–576. [CrossRef] [PubMed]
29. Sleifer, P.; Didoné, D.D.; Keppeler, Í.B.; Bueno, C.D.; Riesgo, R.D.S. Air and Bone Conduction Frequency-specific Auditory Brainstem Response in Children with Agenesis of the External Auditory Canal. *Int. Arch. Otorhinolaryngol.* **2017**, *21*, 318–322. [CrossRef] [PubMed]
30. Gazia, F.; Galletti, B.; Portelli, D.; Alberti, G.; Freni, F.; Bruno, R.; Galletti, F. Real ear measurement (REM) and auditory performances with open, tulip and double closed dome in patients using hearing aids. *Eur. Arch. Otorhinolaryngol.* **2020**, *277*, 1289–1295. [CrossRef] [PubMed]
31. Shimokura, R.; Hosoi, H.; Nishimura, T.; Iwakura, T.; Yamanaka, T. Simulating cartilage conduction sound to estimate the sound pressure level in the external auditory canal. *J. Sound. Vib.* **2015**, *20*, 261–268. [CrossRef]
32. Shimokura, R.; Nishimura, T.; Hosoi, H. Vibrational and Acoustical Characteristics of Ear Pinna Simulators that Differ in Hardness. *Audiol. Res.* **2021**, *11*, 327–334, in press. [CrossRef]

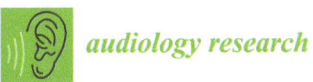

Article

Benefits of Cartilage Conduction Hearing Aids for Speech Perception in Unilateral Aural Atresia

Sakie Akasaka [1], Tadashi Nishimura [1,*], Hiroshi Hosoi [2], Osamu Saito [1], Ryota Shimokura [3], Chihiro Morimoto [1] and Tadashi Kitahara [1]

1. Department of Otolaryngology-Head and Neck Surgery, Nara Medical University, 840 Shijo-cho, Kashihara, Nara 634-8522, Japan; sakasaka@kcn.jp (S.A.); o-saito@naramed-u.ac.jp (O.S.); mori-chi@naramed-u.ac.jp (C.M.); tkitahara@naramed-u.ac.jp (T.K.)
2. MBT (Medicine-Based Town) Institute, Nara Medical University, 840 Shijo-cho, Kashihara, Nara 634-8522, Japan; hosoi@naramed-u.ac.jp
3. Graduate School of Engineering Science, Osaka University, D436, 1-3 Machikaneyama, Toyonaka, Osaka 560-8531, Japan; rshimo@sys.es.osaka-u.ac.jp
* Correspondence: t-nishim@naramed-u.ac.jp; Tel.: +81-744-22-3051

Abstract: Severe conductive hearing loss due to unilateral aural atresia leads to auditory and developmental disorders, such as difficulty in hearing in challenging situations. Bone conduction devices compensate for the disability but unfortunately have several disadvantages. The aim of this study was to evaluate the benefits of cartilage conduction (CC) hearing aids for speech perception in unilateral aural atresia. Eleven patients with unilateral aural atresia were included. Each participant used a CC hearing aid in the atretic ear. Speech recognition scores in the binaural hearing condition were obtained at low speech levels to evaluate the contribution of aided atretic ears to speech perception. Speech recognition scores were also obtained with and without presentation of noise. These assessments were compared between the unaided and aided atretic ear conditions. Speech recognition scores at low speech levels were significantly improved under the aided atretic ear condition ($p < 0.05$). A CC hearing aid in the unilateral atretic ear did not significantly improve the speech recognition score in a symmetrical noise presentation condition. The binaural hearing benefits of CC hearing aids in unilateral aural atresia were predominantly considered a diotic summation. Other benefits of binaural hearing remain to be investigated.

Keywords: atretic ear; unilateral conductive hearing loss; bone conduction; diotic summation; speech recognition

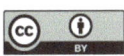

1. Introduction

Unilateral hearing deficit deprives individuals of the benefits of binaural hearing naturally present in individuals with normal hearing and disturbs auditory development [1–4]. Thus, auditory intervention is required for unilateral hearing disability as well as for binaural disability. Representative benefits of binaural hearing are diotic summation, binaural squelch, and improved sound localization [5].

Air conduction (AC) hearing aids are usually used as an intervention device in most individuals with hearing loss. However, some pathological ear conditions, such as atretic ear, prevent the use of AC hearing aids. Bone conduction (BC) hearing aids are effective in atretic ears and are therefore used instead of AC hearing aids in individuals with aural atresia. Unfortunately, BC hearing aids also have several disadvantages concerning comfort, esthetics, and stability [5,6]. Its alternatives include implantable BC devices [7–10], which unfortunately require surgical intervention. For most patients with unilateral aural atresia, these options are not desired.

On attaching a transducer on the aural cartilage, the patient is able to perceive loud sounds [11], and this conduction, termed cartilage conduction (CC), has characteristics different from those of conventional AC and BC [12–16]. CC hearing aids are new, innovative hearing devices utilizing CC, which address the issues concerning the fixation of BC hearing aids and require no surgical intervention [17–21]. Thus, they can be an attractive alternative for patients with unilateral aural atresia.

Hearing via CC is not simple, since both direct-AC sound and airborne sound generated by vibrating the cartilaginous portion of the ear canal result in sound perception [22]. CC hearing provides excessive low-frequency boost depending on the ear conditions [23], which can deteriorate speech perception [24]. However, appropriate gain-adjustment can improve it [25], and according to the previous reports on CC hearing aids, patients with aural atresia had good speech recognition in the aided condition [20]. In Japan, CC hearing aids have been clinically used since 2017 and gained popularity among patients with aural atresia [26–28]. A nationwide clinical survey revealed excellent outcomes of CC hearing aids in the patients who experienced difficulty with AC hearing aids due to aural atresia, canal stenosis, and chronic continuous otorrhea [29].

In clinical use, patients who tried CC hearing aids reported benefits, such as improved conversation in noisy situations and improved sound localization, and they wished to continue using them [20]. Our previous study revealed improved sound localization with CC hearing aid use in patients with bilateral aural atresia [30]. In contrast, the benefits of CC hearing aid in unilateral aural atresia remain unclear. Unilateral aural atresia causes unilateral severe conductive hearing loss, since the patient is deprived of unilateral AC due to a lack of the ear canal. Amplification in the ear affected by unilateral severe hearing loss with a hearing aid improves binaural hearing, which contributes to improved speech recognition, conversation in noisy situations, and sound localization [31,32]. It remains to be investigated whether these binaural hearing benefits are provided with a CC hearing aid in the unilateral atretic ear. The purpose of this study was to clarify the audiological benefits of CC hearing aids for the unilateral atretic ear. The contributions of CC hearing aid to speech perception by the unilateral atretic ear were investigated.

2. Materials and Methods

All participants were recruited from a previous clinical trial of CC hearing aids [20]. Eleven participants (three females; eight males) with unilateral aural atresia who used CC hearing aids were enrolled in the present study. The median age of the participants was 29 years (range, 7–83 years). The average AC and BC hearing levels at 500, 1000, and 2000 Hz in pure tone audiometry of atretic ears were 68.9 ± 15.9 dB and 17.7 ± 8.7 dB, respectively. The average AC for unaffected ears was 14.7 ± 10.8 dB. The study was approved by the ethics committee of Nara Medical University (No. 09-KEN011). Participants provided written informed consent before being enrolled. If the participant's age was <20 years, the parents provided consent.

The average threshold at 500, 1000, and 2000 Hz in atretic ears aided with a CC hearing aid was 35.6 ± 9.0 dB. When the thresholds in the atretic ear were measured in the sound field, normal ear was masked with narrow band noise. In some participants, adequate masker level could not be determined using a plateau method due to a large difference between the two ears, and the unaided threshold in the atretic ear (and functional gain) could not be obtained. Judging from the aided threshold and functional gain in bilateral atretic ears in the previous study, the functional gains for the participants were estimated to be 30–40 dB [20]. The duration of CC hearing aid use was 36.8 ± 11.2 months, while nobody had used other hearing devices before the fitting. The CC hearing aids used in this study were equipped with the directional mode and noise suppression functions. However, these functions had not been activated both for daily use and during the measurement in all subjects.

2.1. Measurement of Speech Recognition at Low Speech Levels

The contribution of CC hearing aids in atretic ears to speech recognition was estimated. The normal ears allowed conversation in quiet environments. The contribution of CC hearing aids in quiet situations is difficult to estimate at more than a moderate speech level. Speech recognition scores were obtained at low speech levels under the unaided and aided conditions, and the scores were compared. In Japan, speech audiometry is conducted using 57-S or 67-S word lists including 50- or 20-monosyllable words, respectively. They are authorized by the Japan Audiological Society [33]. In order to evaluate speech recognition in detail, 57-S word lists are preferable as the test material owing to the larger number of the monosyllables. However, a long examination time is required for the repeated measurements using 57-S word lists. To reduce the burden of the examination, speech performance-intensity functions were first measured using 67-S word lists. Speech recognition was measured in 10-dB steps under the unaided condition. The speech level at which the maximum score was obtained in the speech performance-intensity function was defined as the "dB (Max)". After the dB (Max) was determined using 67-S word lists for each participant, speech recognition tests using the 57-S word lists were conducted under the unaided and aided conditions. The measurements were conducted not only at the dB (Max), but also at 10 dB below the dB (Max), which was defined as the "dB (Max-10)." In this study, dB (Max-10) was employed as a low speech level. The determination procedures of the dB (Max) and dB (Max-10) are described in Figure 1.

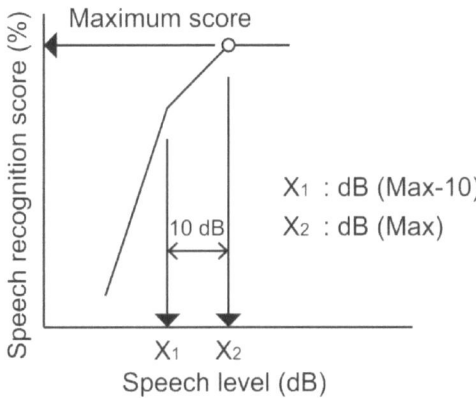

Figure 1. Determination of the dB (Max) and dB (Max-10). Speech performance-intensity function under the unaided binaural hearing condition was measured using 20-monosyllable word lists in 10-dB steps. The minimum speech level at which the maximum speech recognition score was obtained was termed the "dB (Max)" (X_2 in the figure); the "dB (Max-10)" was determined by subtracting 10 dB from the dB (Max) (X_1 in the figure).

2.2. Measurement of Speech Recognition in Noise

The speech recognition scores with and without noise were compared under the unaided and aided conditions. A loudspeaker for speech presentation was located 1 m in front of each participant. Two loudspeakers for noise presentation were individually located at ±45 degrees azimuth at a distance of 1 m according to ISO 8253-3 (2012). The 57-S word lists and speech-weighted noise were employed as the test material and noise, respectively. The power spectrum of the speech-weighted noise was constant from 125 Hz to 1000 Hz, with a roll-off of 12 dB/oct [34]. The presented noise between two loudspeakers was uncorrelated. Speech recognition scores were obtained at a 60-dB hearing level in the unaided and aided binaural hearing conditions, and the measurements were performed with and without noise presentation. The signal-to-noise ratio (SNR) was set at +10 dB. These procedures were performed according to guidelines that are standard in Japan [35].

The above-mentioned assessments were performed in a soundproof room (dimensions, approximately 5.4 m × 5.4 m). The calibration of the loudspeakers was carried out with a sound level meter (NA-20; Rion, Kokubunji, Japan).

2.3. Statistical Analysis

Speech recognition scores at two speech levels were analyzed using two-way analysis of variance (ANOVA), with hearing aid (aided with CC hearing aid or not) and speech levels as within-subject factors. The impact of noise on speech recognition scores were also analyzed using two-way ANOVA, with hearing aid and noise (with and without noise presentation) as within-subject factors. Statistical ANOVA was performed using SPSS ver. 22 (International Business Machines Corporation, Armonk, NY, USA). The Bonferroni method was used as a post-hoc correction of the multiple comparisons test after ANOVA. Significance was set at 0.05.

3. Results

The obtained speech performance-intensity functions determined the dB (Max) of each participant. The average dB (Max) was 35.4 ± 12.1 dB. Figure 2A shows the speech recognition scores at the dB (Max) and dB (Max-10) under the unaided and aided conditions. ANOVA revealed a significant effect for speech level ($F(10, 1) = 37.57, p < 0.01$), but not for the hearing aid ($F(10, 1) = 3.07, p = 0.11$). A significant interaction between them was found ($F(10, 1) = 7.54, p < 0.05$). In the post-hoc tests at the dB (Max-10), the speech recognition score under the aided condition was found to be $54.0 \pm 20.0\%$, which was significantly higher than that under the unaided condition, which was $44.7 \pm 19.4\%$ ($p < 0.05$).

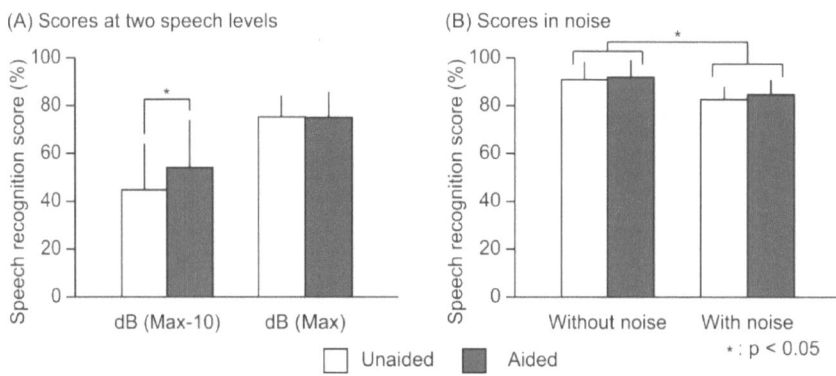

Figure 2. Speech recognition scores at two speech levels (**A**) and with/without noise presentation (**B**). Speech recognition scores were measured using 50-monosyllable word lists in unaided and aided binaural hearing conditions. Vertical bars indicate standard deviations.

The speech recognition scores decreased under the noise presentation condition (Figure 2B). ANOVA revealed a significant effect for noise ($F(10, 1) = 12.20, p < 0.01$), but not for the hearing aid ($F(10, 1) = 1.56, p = 0.24$). No interaction between them was found ($F(10, 1) = 0.14, p = 0.72$). Speech recognition scores significantly decreased with noise presentation. No differences in the decrease were found between the unaided and aided conditions.

4. Discussion

The benefits of CC hearing aids in unilateral aural atresia were evaluated. We investigated the effects of a CC hearing aid in the atretic ear on speech recognition at low speech levels and in presence of noise. Only the benefit of diotic summation on speech recognition was obtained in this study.

Unilateral aural atresia induces severe conductive hearing loss of the atretic ear, which causes a large difference between the two ears. The amplification gain with CC hearing aids is estimated to be 30–40 dB [20], reducing the left–right difference in hearing. This study tried to evaluate the contribution of CC hearing aids in atretic ears to speech recognition. When the presentation level is high enough for the normal ear alone to accurately understand the speech, the contribution of the atretic ear cannot be detected. Therefore, the speech recognition scores under the unaided and aided conditions were obtained at 2 presentation levels: dB (Max) and dB (Max-10). Although no difference in speech recognition scores was observed at the dB (Max), binaural hearing benefit on speech recognition was observed at the dB (max-10). Low speech level condition revealed the contribution of the aided atretic ear to speech recognition. Diotic summation contributes to improving speech recognition in difficult hearing conditions [36]. The sound condition in daily conversation is poorer than that in the experimental room. CC hearing aids in atretic ears are expected to assist real-life listening by the diotic summation.

Another advantage of binaural hearing is improved hearing in noisy situations. Individuals with binaural hearing can benefit from head shadow effects just by attending to the ear with the better SNR [37]. Furthermore, the auditory system can combine different mixtures of speech and noise arriving at each ear to effectively remove some of the noise [38]. Unfortunately, no binaural hearing benefit was identified in this study. The reduction of speech intelligibility due to noise has been associated with various factors, including localization of noise, SNR, and type of noise [39,40]. Speech-weighted noises were presented from ±45 degrees azimuth according to ISO 8253-3 (2012), which symmetrically disturbed the hearing in both ears. In such a noise presentation condition, binaural squelch did not function well. In previous studies, the speech recognition under noise condition was improved with a bone anchored hearing aid (BAHA) in the atretic side [41,42]. However, those evaluations were conducted with different arrangements of signal and noise presentation. They placed the loudspeakers for noise presentation contralateral to the BAHA side. In this noise presentation condition, binaural squelch provided its benefits. If the current measurements were conducted in similar noise presentation condition as these previous studies, the benefits would be observed.

Limitations of the Study

Most patients with unilateral aural atresia who have tried CC hearing aids in atretic ears wished to continuously use the aids, as they subjectively perceived the benefits of binaural hearing after daily use [20]. This study evaluated the benefits of binaural hearing in terms of speech recognition and speech recognition under noise presentation. However, significant improvement was objectively observed only for speech recognition at low speech levels. The other factors such as age and laterality probably influence the benefits of binaural hearing. The sample size of this study was too small to determine the impact of these factors. In terms of the experimental condition, the arrangement of loudspeakers and the type of noise present have to be reconsidered. Further study is required to elucidate the benefits of CC hearing aids in a unilateral atretic ear.

5. Conclusions

The benefits of binaural hearing with CC hearing aids in unilateral aural atresia were evaluated. By decreasing the left–right difference in hearing, speech recognition scores improved at low speech levels. No improvements in speech recognition in noise were found. The binaural hearing benefits of CC hearing aids in unilateral aural atresia were predominantly considered to be a diotic summation.

Author Contributions: Conceptualization, S.A., T.N., O.S., and C.M.; statistical analysis, T.N. and R.S.; investigation, S.A., and T.N.; data curation, T.N., and O.S.; writing—original draft preparation, S.A., and T.N.; writing—review and editing, H.H.; Approval of the manuscript: H.H., and T.K.; funding acquisition, C.M. All authors have read and agreed to the published version of the manuscript.

Funding: This research was supported by JSPS KAKENHI Grant Number 17K11339 and 19K09874, and also supported by the Japan Agency for Medical Research and Development (AMED), grant number 15he1302011g0003.

Institutional Review Board Statement: The study was conducted according to the guidelines of the Declaration of Helsinki, and approved by the ethics committee of Nara Medical University (No. 09-KEN011).

Informed Consent Statement: Participants provided written informed consent before being enrolled. If the participant's age was <20 years, the parents provided consent.

Data Availability Statement: Not applicable.

Conflicts of Interest: Cartilage conduction hearing aids were manufactured and supplied by Rion Co., Ltd., Kokubunji, Tokyo, Japan for a previous clinical study [20].

References

1. Huttunen, K.; Erixon, E.; Löfkvist, U.; Mäki-Torkko, E. The impact of permanent early-onset unilateral hearing impairment in children—A systematic review. *Int. J. Pediatr. Otorhinolaryngol.* **2019**, *120*, 173–183. [CrossRef] [PubMed]
2. Bagatto, M.; DesGeorges, J.; King, A.; Kitterick, P.; Laurnagaray, D.; Lewis, D.; Roush, P.; Sladen, D.P.; Tharpe, A.M. Consensus practice parameter: Audiological assessment and management of unilateral hearing loss in children. *Int. J. Audiol.* **2019**, *58*, 805–815. [CrossRef] [PubMed]
3. Gordon, K.; Kral, A. Animal and human studies on developmental monaural hearing loss. *Hear. Res.* **2019**, *380*, 60–74. [CrossRef]
4. Yang, F.; Zheng, Y.; Li, G. Early prelingual auditory development of infants and toddlers with unilateral hearing loss. *Otol. Neurotol.* **2020**, *41*, 650–654. [CrossRef]
5. Dillon, H. *Hearing Aids*; Thieme: Stuttgart, Germany, 2001.
6. Lo, J.F.; Tsang, W.S.; Yu, J.Y.; Ho, O.Y.; Ku, P.K.; Tong, M.C. Contemporary hearing rehabilitation options in patients with aural atresia. *BioMed Res. Int.* **2014**, *2014*, 761579. [CrossRef] [PubMed]
7. Ikeda, R.; Hidaka, H.; Murata, T.; Miyazaki, H.; Katori, Y.; Kobayashi, T. Vibrant Soundbridge implantation via a retrofacial approach in a patient with congenital aural atresia. *Auris Nasus Larynx* **2019**, *46*, 204–209. [CrossRef]
8. Håkansson, B.; Reinfeldt, S.; Persson, A.C.; Jansson, K.F.; Rigato, C.; Hultcrantz, M.; Eeg-Olofsson, M. The bone conduction implant—A review and 1-year follow-up. *Int. J. Audiol.* **2019**, *58*, 945–955. [CrossRef]
9. Oh, S.J.; Goh, E.K.; Choi, S.W.; Lee, S.; Lee, H.M.; Lee, I.W.; Kong, S.K. Audiologic, surgical and subjective outcomes of active transcutaneous bone conduction implant system (Bonebridge). *Int. J. Audiol.* **2019**, *58*, 956–963. [CrossRef] [PubMed]
10. Curca, I.A.; Parsa, V.; Macpherson, E.A.; Scollie, S.; Vansevenant, K.; Zimmerman, K.; Lewis-Teeter, J.; Allen, P.; Parnes, L.; Agrawal, S. Audiological outcome measures with the BONEBRIDGE transcutaneous bone conduction hearing implant: Impact of noise, reverberation and signal processing features. *Int. J. Audiol.* **2020**, *59*, 556–565. [CrossRef]
11. Shimokura, R.; Hosoi, H.; Nishimura, T.; Yamanaka, T.; Levitt, H. Cartilage conduction hearing. *J. Acoust. Soc. Am.* **2014**, *135*, 1959–1966. [CrossRef]
12. Nishimura, T.; Hosoi, H.; Saito, O.; Miyamae, R.; Shimokura, R.; Matsui, T.; Yamanaka, T.; Levitt, H. Is cartilage conduction classified into air or bone conduction? *Laryngoscope* **2014**, *124*, 1214–1219. [CrossRef]
13. Nishimura, T.; Hosoi, H.; Saito, O.; Miyamae, R.; Shimokura, R.; Yamanaka, T.; Kitahara, T.; Levitt, H. Cartilage conduction is characterized by vibrations of the cartilaginous portion of the ear canal. *PLoS ONE* **2015**, *10*, e0120135. [CrossRef]
14. Nishimura, T.; Hosoi, H.; Saito, O.; Miyamae, R.; Shimokura, R.; Matsui, T.; Yamanaka, T.; Levitt, H. Cartilage conduction efficiently generates airborne sound in the ear canal. *Auris Nasus Larynx* **2015**, *42*, 15–19. [CrossRef]
15. Hosoi, H.; Nishimura, T.; Shimokura, R.; Kitahara, T. Cartilage conduction as the third pathway for sound transmission. *Auris Nasus Larynx* **2019**, *46*, 151–159. [CrossRef]
16. Nishimura, T.; Hosoi, H.; Saito, O.; Akasaka, S.; Shimokura, R.; Yamanaka, T.; Kitahara, T. Effect of fixation place on airborne sound in cartilage conduction. *J. Acoust. Soc. Am.* **2020**, *148*, 469. [CrossRef] [PubMed]
17. Hosoi, H.; Yanai, S.; Nishimura, T.; Sakaguchi, T.; Iwakura, T.; Yoshino, K. Development of cartilage conduction hearing aid. *Arch. Mat. Sci. Eng.* **2010**, *42*, 104–110.
18. Nishimura, T.; Hosoi, H.; Saito, O.; Miyamae, R.; Shimokura, R.; Matsui, T.; Iwakura, T. Benefit of a new hearing device utilizing cartilage conduction. *Auris Nasus Larynx* **2013**, *40*, 440–446. [CrossRef]
19. Shimokura, R.; Hosoi, H.; Iwakura, T.; Nishimura, T.; Matsui, T. Development of monaural and binaural behind-the-ear cartilage conduction hearing aids. *Appl. Acoust.* **2013**, *74*, 1234–1240. [CrossRef]
20. Nishimura, T.; Hosoi, H.; Saito, O.; Shimokura, R.; Yamanaka, T.; Kitahara, T. Cartilage Conduction Hearing Aids for Severe Conduction Hearing Loss. *Otol. Neurotol.* **2018**, *39*, 65–72. [CrossRef] [PubMed]
21. Nishimura, T.; Hosoi, H.; Shimokura, R.; Morimoto, C.; Kitahara, T. Cartilage Conduction Hearing and Its Clinical Application. *Audiol. Res.* **2021**, *11*, 23. [CrossRef]
22. Shimokura, R.; Hosoi, H.; Nishimura, T.; Iwakura, T.; Yamanaka, T. Simulating cartilage conduction sound to estimate the sound pressure level in the external auditory canal. *J. Sound Vib.* **2015**, *20*, 261–268. [CrossRef]
23. Morimoto, C.; Nishimura, T.; Hosoi, H.; Saito, O.; Fukuda, F.; Shimokura, R.; Yamanaka, T. Sound transmission by cartilage conduction in ear with fibrotic aural atresia. *J. Rehabil. Res. Dev.* **2014**, *51*, 325–332. [CrossRef]

24. Miyamae, R.; Nishimura, T.; Hosoi, H.; Saito, O.; Shimokura, R.; Yamanaka, T.; Kitahara, T. Perception of speech in cartilage conduction. *Auris Nasus Larynx* **2017**, *44*, 26–32. [CrossRef]
25. Nishimura, T.; Miyamae, R.; Hosoi, H.; Saito, O.; Shimokura, R.; Yamanaka, T.; Kitahara, T. Frequency characteristics and speech recognition in cartilage conduction. *Auris Nasus Larynx* **2019**, *46*, 709–715. [CrossRef] [PubMed]
26. Sakamoto, Y.; Shimada, A.; Nakano, S.; Kondo, E.; Takeyama, T.; Fukuda, J.; Udaka, J.; Okamoto, H.; Takeda, N. Effects of FM system fitted into the normal hearing ear or cartilage conduction hearing aid fitted into the affected ear on speech-in-noise recognition in Japanese children with unilateral congenital aural atresia. *J. Med. Investig.* **2020**, *67*, 131–138. [CrossRef]
27. Nishiyama, T.; Oishi, N.; Ogawa, K. Who are good adult candidates for cartilage conduction hearing aids? *Eur. Arch. Otorhinolaryngol.* **2020**, in press. [CrossRef]
28. Nishiyama, T.; Oishi, N.; Ogawa, K. Efficacy of cartilage conduction hearing aids in children. *Int. J. Pediatr. Otorhinolaryngol.* **2021**, *142*, 110628. [CrossRef]
29. Nishimura, T.; Hosoi, H.; Sugiuchi, T.; Matsumoto, N.; Nishiyama, T.; Takano, K.; Sugimoto, S.; Yazama, H.; Sato, T.; Komori, M. Cartilage conduction hearing aid fitting in clinical practice. *J. Am. Acad. Audiol.* **2021**, in press. [CrossRef]
30. Nishimura, T.; Hosoi, H.; Saito, O.; Shimokura, R.; Yamanaka, T.; Kitahara, T. Sound localisation ability using cartilage conduction hearing aids in bilateral aural atresia. *Int. J. Audiol.* **2020**, *59*, 891–896. [CrossRef] [PubMed]
31. Johnstone, P.M.; Nábělek, A.K.; Robertson, V.S. Sound localization acuity in children with unilateral hearing loss who wear a hearing aid in the impaired ear. *J. Am. Acad. Audiol.* **2010**, *21*, 522–534. [CrossRef] [PubMed]
32. Bishop, C.E.; Hamadain, E.; Galster, J.A.; Johnson, M.F.; Spankovich, C.; Windmill, I. Outcomes of Hearing Aid Use by Individuals with Unilateral Sensorineural Hearing Loss (USNHL). *J. Am. Acad. Audiol.* **2017**, *28*, 941–949. [CrossRef]
33. Japan Audiological Society. Methods of speech audiometry. *Audiol. Japan.* **2003**, *46*, 621–637. [CrossRef]
34. Nishimura, T.; Okayasu, T.; Saito, O.; Shimokura, R.; Yamashita, A.; Yamanaka, T.; Hosoi, H.; Kitahara, T. An examination of the effects of broadband air-conduction masker on the speech intelligibility of speech-modulated bone-conduction ultrasound. *Hear. Res.* **2014**, *317*, 41–49. [CrossRef]
35. Kodera, K.; Hosoi, H.; Okamoto, M.; Manabe, T.; Kanda, Y.; Shiraishi, K.; Sugiuchi, T.; Suzuki, K.; Tauchi, H.; Nishimura, T.; et al. Guidelines for the evaluation of hearing aid fitting (2010). *Auris Nasus Larynx* **2016**, *43*, 217–228. [CrossRef]
36. Davis, A.; Haggard, M.; Bell, I. Magnitude of diotic summation in speech-in-noise tasks: Performance region and appropriate baseline. *Br. J. Audiol.* **1990**, *24*, 11–16. [CrossRef]
37. Schoenmaker, E.; Sutojo, S.; van de Par, S. Better-ear rating based on glimpsing. *J. Acoust. Soc. Am.* **2017**, *142*, 1466. [CrossRef]
38. Hilly, O.; Sokolov, M.; Finkel, R.B.; Zavdy, O.; Shemesh, R.; Attias, J. Hearing in noise with unilateral versus bilateral bone conduction hearing aids in adults with pseudo-conductive hearing loss. *Otol. Neurotol.* **2020**, *41*, 379–385. [CrossRef] [PubMed]
39. Weisser, A.; Buchholz, J.M. Conversational speech levels and signal-to-noise ratios in realistic acoustic conditions. *J. Acoust. Soc. Am.* **2019**, *145*, 349. [CrossRef]
40. Wagner, L.; Geiling, L.; Hauth, C.; Hocke, T.; Plontke, S.; Rahne, T. Improved binaural speech reception thresholds through small symmetrical separation of speech and noise. *PLoS ONE* **2020**, *15*, e0236469. [CrossRef]
41. Hol, M.K.; Snik, A.F.; Mylanus, E.A.; Cremers, C.W. Does the bone-anchored hearing aid have a complementary effect on audiological and subjective outcomes in patients with unilateral conductive hearing loss? *Audiol. Neurootol.* **2005**, *10*, 159–168. [CrossRef]
42. Kunst, S.J.; Leijendeckers, J.M.; Mylanus, E.A.; Hol, M.K.; Snik, A.F.; Cremers, C.W. Bone-anchored hearing aid system application for unilateral congenital conductive hearing impairment: Audiometric results. *Otol. Neurotol.* **2008**, *29*, 2–7. [CrossRef] [PubMed]

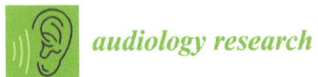

Article

Management of Residual Hearing with Cartilage Conduction Hearing Aid after Lateral Temporal Bone Resection: Our Institutional Experience

Noritaka Komune [1,*], Yoshie Higashino [1], Kazuha Ishikawa [1], Tomoko Tabuki [1], Shogo Masuda [1], Kensuke Koike [1], Takahiro Hongo [1], Kuniaki Sato [1], Ryutaro Uchi [1], Masaru Miyazaki [2], Ryo Shimamoto [3], Nana Akagi Tsuchihashi [1], Ryunosuke Kogo [1], Teppei Noda [1], Nozomu Matsumoto [1] and Takashi Nakagawa [1]

1. Department of Otorhinolaryngology, Graduate School of Medical Sciences, Kyushu University, Fukuoka 812-8582, Japan; y-hgsn@qent.med.kyushu-u.ac.jp (Y.H.); horikiri@med.kyushu-u.ac.jp (K.I.); tabuki@med.kyushu-u.ac.jp (T.T.); shogo.masuda117@gmail.com (S.M.); kensuke11242000@gmail.com (K.K.); orihakat.ognoh@gmail.com (T.H.); basement.kuni13@gmail.com (K.S.); urentcello@gmail.com (R.U.); nanaakagi0707@yahoo.co.jp (N.A.T.); ryukogo@gmail.com (R.K.); teppei@med.kyushu-u.ac.jp (T.N.); matsumoto.nozomu.297@m.kyushu-u.ac.jp (N.M.); nakataka@med.kyushu-u.ac.jp (T.N.)
2. Department of Otorhinolaryngology, Fukuoka University Hospital and School of Medicine, Fukuoka 812-8582, Japan; masarumiyazaki@fukuoka-u.ac.jp
3. Department of Plastic Surgery, Graduate School of Medical Sciences, Kyushu University, Fukuoka 812-8582, Japan; say.hello.to.ryo@gmail.com
* Correspondence: norikomu007@gmail.com; Tel.: +81-92-642-5668

Abstract: Background: There is no guideline for hearing compensation after temporal bone resection. This study aimed to retrospectively analyze surgical cases with reconstruction for hearing preservation after temporal bone malignancy resection and propose a new alternative to compensate for hearing loss. Methods: We retrospectively reviewed the medical records of 30 patients who underwent lateral temporal bone surgery for temporal bone malignancy at our institution and examined their hearing abilities after surgery. Result: The hearing outcomes of patients with an external auditory meatus reconstruction varied widely. The mean postoperative air–bone gap at 0.5, 1, 2, and 4 kHz ranged from 22.5 dB to 71.25 dB. On the other hand, the average difference between the aided sound field thresholds with cartilage conduction hearing aid and bone conduction thresholds at 0.5, 1, 2, and 4 kHz ranged from −3.75 to 41.25. More closely located auricular cartilage and temporal bone resulted in smaller differences between the aided sound field and bone conduction thresholds. Conclusions: There is still room for improvement of surgical techniques for reconstruction of the auditory meatus to preserve hearing after temporal bone resection. The cartilage conduction hearing aid may provide non-invasive postoperative hearing compensation after lateral temporal bone resection.

Keywords: temporal bone resection; hearing management; cartilage conduction hearing aid

1. Introduction

Malignant tumors of the temporal bone are rare with an extremely low incidence rate [1,2]. The most common histological type is squamous cell carcinoma, followed by adenoid cystic carcinoma. Currently, the establishment of clinical evidence is slow due to the rarity of this entity. In the existing literature, negative margin resection has been recognized to some extent as the standard of treatment. However, there is currently no global consensus on the treatment protocol.

Additionally, each facility may have various treatment strategies to compensate for hearing loss after temporal bone resection. Patients with temporal bone malignancies are often provided with treatment options that result in hearing loss. Hearing loss leads to the deterioration of patients' quality of life. To compensate, hearing improvement after surgery is desirable, but there is no standard protocol or guideline on this issue.

It has been shown that negative margin resection for temporal bone malignancies provides excellent long-term tumor-free survival. While the use of hearing preservation surgery with auditory canal reconstruction and tympanoplasty after temporal bone resection has recently been reported, surgical results remain under discussion and in need of improvement. Morita et al. reported favorable results in eight cases of auditory canal reconstruction using split-thickness skin grafts for surgically treated early temporal bone malignancies [3]. However, few reports have detailed postoperative hearing results [3,4].

Nishimura's group first introduced cartilage conduction hearing in clinical practice. A cartilage conduction hearing aid (CCHA) includes both the cartilage–bone sound pathway and the cartilage–air and direct air pathway. This small and non-invasive device was considered as an option for hearing compensation after lateral temporal bone surgery [5–10].

In this report, to discuss options for hearing compensation after lateral temporal bone resection (LTBR), we report the postoperative hearing progression of cases with external auditory canal reconstruction after lateral temporal bone resection (LTBR) and the results of our examination of the effectiveness of the CCHA after LTBR.

2. Material and Methods

2.1. Patient Selection

A retrospective review of the patients treated at the Department of Otorhinolaryngology, Head and Neck Surgery at the Kyushu University Hospital from January 1993 to July 2020 was performed. A total of 181 patients were treated for temporal bone-related malignancies. A total of 161 cases of malignancies originated from the temporal bone. LTBR cases with postoperative hearing compensation were selected for this review. The final dataset included nine patients who underwent LTBR with the reconstruction of the external auditory meatus and tympanoplasty. Furthermore, we obtained audiometric data from 16 cases aided with CCHAs. Approval from the ethics review committee of Kyushu University Hospital (permit no. 29–43) was obtained.

2.2. Treatment Strategy for Temporal Bone Squamous Cell Carcinoma at Our Institute

All patients with temporal bone squamous cell carcinoma were treated with LTBR. When a postoperative pathological examination revealed a positive resection margin or if it was highly suspected intraoperatively, postoperative chemoradiotherapy was added. When the tumor was considered resectable with free negative margins on preoperative computed tomography (CT) and magnetic resonance imaging (MRI) scans, reconstruction of the external auditory canal with a free flap was planned for the patient undergoing hearing-preserving surgery.

2.3. Audiometric Data

Audiometry with a pure-tone audiometer (AA-76, AA-78, AA-79; Rion, Kokubunji, Japan) was conducted in a soundproof booth by experienced audiologists. Pure-tone thresholds were measured at 0.125, 0.25, 0.5, 1, 2, 4, and 8 kHz frequencies for air conduction and at 0.25, 0.5, 1, 2, 4 kHz for bone conduction with masking as appropriate. The results of both preoperative and postoperative hearing thresholds are included in our dataset. The hearing level was evaluated based on pure-tone audiograms as a follow-up to postoperative hearing levels in patients with auditory canal reconstruction. Pure-tone air and bone conduction thresholds averages were obtained. For pure-tone averages, the thresholds measured were 0.5, 1, 2, and 4 kHz. Air-bone gaps (ABGs) were calculated using air and bone conduction averages from the same test. To test the hearing level in patients that underwent surgery with the bone–cartilage anchoring technique, ipsilateral pure-tone hearing thresholds were tested while the patients wore commercial CCHAs (HB-J1CC, Rion) with appropriate masking for the contralateral side. We calculated and averaged the difference between the aided sound field thresholds and bone conduction thresholds at 0.5, 1, 2, and 4 kHz, which is referred to as "aided ABG."

2.4. Image Analysis

An axial image of CT was used to measure the closest distance between the auricular cartilage and temporal bone after surgery.

3. Results

3.1. Patient Profile

Our study included 30 patients that underwent LTBR, among which nine cases underwent the reconstruction of the external auditory meatus and tympanoplasty and 12 cases underwent the closure of the external auditory meatus. Five out of 12 cases underwent LTBR with the bone–cartilage anchoring technique to establish firm contact between the cartilage and the temporal bone. We obtained audiometric data from 16 cases aided with CCHAs after surgery. Pathology, clinical T stage (based on the modified Pittsburgh classification), sex, age, affected side, type of surgical approach, type of free flap for reconstruction, operation time, surgeon, resection margin examination, adjuvant radiotherapy, and aided ABG are summarized in Table 1. In cases 11 and 13, tumor invasion of the resected margin was highly suspected intraoperatively; for this reason, postoperative radiotherapy was added, although surgical margins were reported as free of carcinoma. In case 15 and 20, postoperative radiotherapy was added because of the extranodal extension. Case 8 and 10 purchased the hearing aid after surgery. The rest of the patients decided not to purchase the hearing aid yet, because their hearing level on the contralateral side was still adequate.

3.2. Reconstruction of the External Auditory Meatus with a Free Flap and Hearing Outcome

The surgical steps for the reconstruction of the external auditory meatus with a free flap are shown in Figure 1. After the en bloc LTBR was done, an anterolateral thigh flap (Cases 1–5, 7 and 9) or groin flap (Cases 6 and 8) with a vascular pedicle was elevated. The skin island flap for the tympanic membrane and auditory meatus was prepared and rolled (Figure 1A). For the tympanic membrane, the subcutaneous tissue was removed to produce a thin layer of vascularized skin. The rolled flap was placed into the temporal bone defect. At the same time, the skin of the tympanic membrane was attached to the bony or cartilage columella on the stapes head (type III tympanoplasty) (Figure 1B). Preoperative and 1-year postoperative pure-tone audiometry results and the reconstructed external auditory meatus in a representative case are shown in Figure 1C,D.

The postoperative follow-up for hearing levels was reviewed in all nine patients with external auditory canal reconstruction. Mean postoperative air–bone gap varied from 22.5 dB to 71.25 dB (Figure 2A). At 2 kHz, the postoperative ABG was at a minimum and varied from 10 dB to 60 dB (Figure 2B).

Postoperative air conduction level also varied from 25 dB to 90 dB at 0.5 Hz, from 30 dB to 95 dB at 1 kHz, from 45 dB to 110 dB at 2 kHz, and from 65 dB to 115 dB at 4 kHz (Figure 2C). The auditory meatus was preserved in eight out of nine patients. In case 6, the volume of the free flap was too great to maintain the structure of the auditory canal and resulted in stenosis of the auditory meatus, which ensued in a mean postoperative ABG of 71.25 dB. This patient was in the process of planning an additional surgery to reduce the volume of the flap and conserve the external auditory meatus.

Table 1. Case profiles.

#	Pathology	cT	Sex	Age	Side	Approach	Reconstruction	Ope Time	Surgeon ENT	Surgeon Plastic	Margin	PORT	(Gy)	BCA	Aided ABG (dB)
With EAC reconstruction															
1	w-m SCC	1	F	74	R	LTBR	ALT	9 h 22 min	NM	SY	−	−	0	−	
2	w-m SCC	1	M	62	R	LTBR	ALT	10 h 26 min	TN/NM	KK	−	−	0	−	
3	w SCC	1	F	61	R	LTBR	ALT	10 h 19 min	NM	RS/SY	+	+	60	−	
4	w SCC	1	F	78	R	LTBR	ALT	6 h 41 min	NM	SY	−	−	0	−	
5	w SCC	4	F	72	R	LTBR	ALT	10 h 41 min	NK	RS	+	+	60	−	30
6	w-m SCC	4	F	66	R	LTBR	Groin	9 h 00 min	NK	SY	−	−	0	−	38.75
7	ACC	1	F	83	R	LTBR	ALT	9 h 39 min	NM	SY	−	−	0	−	
8	ACC	2	M	58	R	LTBR	Groin	9 h 53 min	TNo/NK	HK	+	+	60	−	27.5
9	ACC	4	F	76	L	LTBR	ALT	14 h 19 min	TNo/NK	RS	+	+	70	−	−3.75
Without EAC reconstruction															
10	w SCC	4	F	33	R	LTBR	ALT	17 h 57 min	TNo/NK	KI	+	+	60	+	20
11	w-m SCC	2	F	67	R	LTBR	ALT	12 h 44 min	NK	RS/KI	−	+	50	+	11.25
12	w SCC	2	M	56	L	LTBR	PAT	5 h 32 min	NK	RS	−	−	0	+	7.5
13	w SCC	2	F	55	L	LTBR	ALT	8 h 56 min	NK	SY	−	+	60	+	17.5
14	w SCC	4	F	66	L	LTBR	ALT	13 h 8 min	NK	RS	−	−	0	+	36.25
15	w-p SCC	2	F	69	L	LTBR	TM	7 h 30 min	NK	NK	−	+	60	+	30
16	w SCC	4	F	48	L	LTBR	ALT	15 h 38 min	NK	SF	−	+	0	−	41.25
17	w SCC	1	F	68	L	LTBR	ALT	9 h 36 min	NK	HK	−	−	0	−	35
18	w SCC	4	F	60	R	LTBR	ALT	10 h 21 min	NK	KI	−	−	0	−	23.75
19	w SCC	3	F	66	R	LTBR	TM	6 h 31 min	NK	NK	−	−	0	−	13.75
20	w SCC	4	F	71	R	LTBR	ALT	12 h 48 min	NK	CO	−	+	60	−	7.5
21	w SCC	2	M	66	L	LTBR	PAT	6 h 51 min	NK	YI	−	−	0	−	1.25

The difference between the aided sound field thresholds and bone conduction thresholds at 0.5, 1, 2, and 4 kHz were calculated and averaged, which is referred to as "aided ABG." ACC, adenoid cystic carcinoma; ALT, anterolateral thigh; BCA, bone-cartilage anchoring technique; CCHA, cartilage conduction hearing aid; EAC, external auditory canal; LTBR, lateral temporal bone resection; PAT, perifascial areolar tissue; PORT, postoperative radiotherapy; SCC, squamous cell carcinoma; w, well differentiated; w-m, well to moderately differentiated; w-p, well to poorly differentiated.

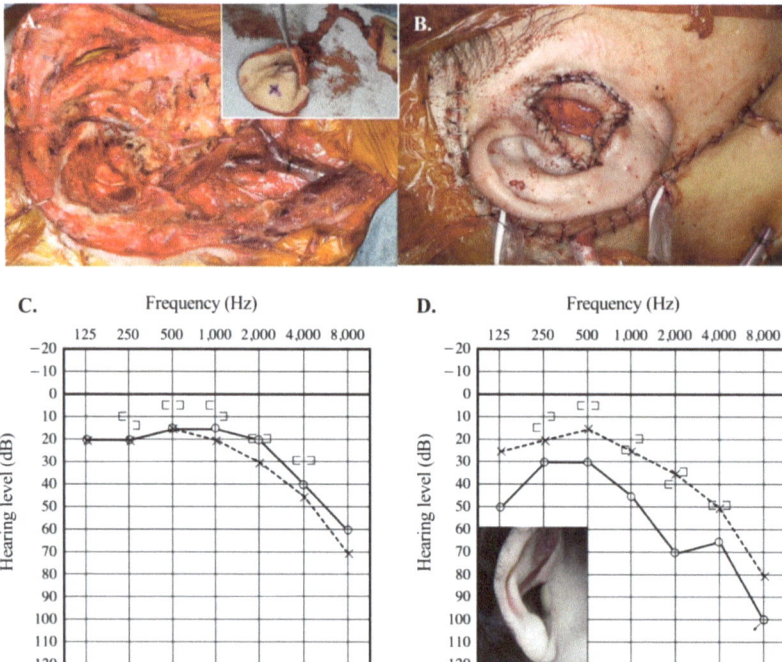

Figure 1. Reconstruction of the external auditory canal after lateral temporal bone resection. (**A**) Surgical view of completed lateral temporal bone resection. An inset shows the harvested free anterolateral thigh flap, which is rolled to create the external auditory meatus. (**B**) Final view after reconstruction of the external auditory meatus. (**C**) Preoperative pure-tone audiometry (Case 1) (**D**) Postoperative pure-tone audiometry one year after surgery (Case 1). Inset shows the reconstructed auditory canal in Case 1.

3.3. Effectiveness of the CCHA

We examined the audiometric data of 16 patients wearing the CCHAs. In four cases with and 12 cases without external auditory reconstruction, we obtained audiometric data postoperatively using the CCHAs. The results showed that the average difference between the aided sound field thresholds and bone conduction thresholds at 0.5, 1, 2, and 4 kHz ranged from −3.75 to 41.25. There was a moderate correlation between the distance between the auricular cartilage and the temporal bone around the triangular fossa and the postoperative difference between the aided sound field thresholds and bone conduction thresholds. Here, the closer the distance, the smaller the difference ($p = 0.0021$ $R2 = 0.503$; Figure 3A). When comparing patients who underwent intraoperative cartilage–bone anchoring with those who did not, treated patients showed lower mean values but with no statistical significance (Figure 3B).

3.4. Bone-Cartilage Anchoring Technique

At our institution, we devised an intraoperative method to establish contact between the cartilage and the bone that increased the effectiveness of the CCHAs in five cases. After LTBR, the cartilage of the triangular fossa is exposed from the wound surface. Two types of anchoring were proposed. The first option is to fix the surface of the triangular fossa cartilage to the temporal bone (Figure 4A,B). The second option is to fix the reflected cartilage of the triangular fossa to the created bony groove at the temporal bone (Figure 4C,D). Preoperative and postoperative hearing levels of a representative patient (Case 3) are shown in Figure 4E,F. Postoperative pure-tone audiometry revealed an apparent conductive hearing loss on the ipsilateral side (Figure 4F). CCHA use improved the hearing level on the ipsilateral side, and the average of the aided sound field threshold with appropriate masking on the contralateral side resulted in 26.25 dB (Figure 4F). For the five patients treated with the bone–cartilage anchoring technique, we calculated the difference between the aided sound field and bone conduction thresholds postoperatively. The average difference at 0.5, 1, 2, and 4 kHz was less than 25 dB postoperatively for the four patients (Figure 5). In case 14, the average difference at 0.5, 1, 2, and 4 kHz was 36.25, but the distance between the auricular cartilage and the temporal bone was largest among cases using the bone–cartilage anchoring technique (Figure 5).

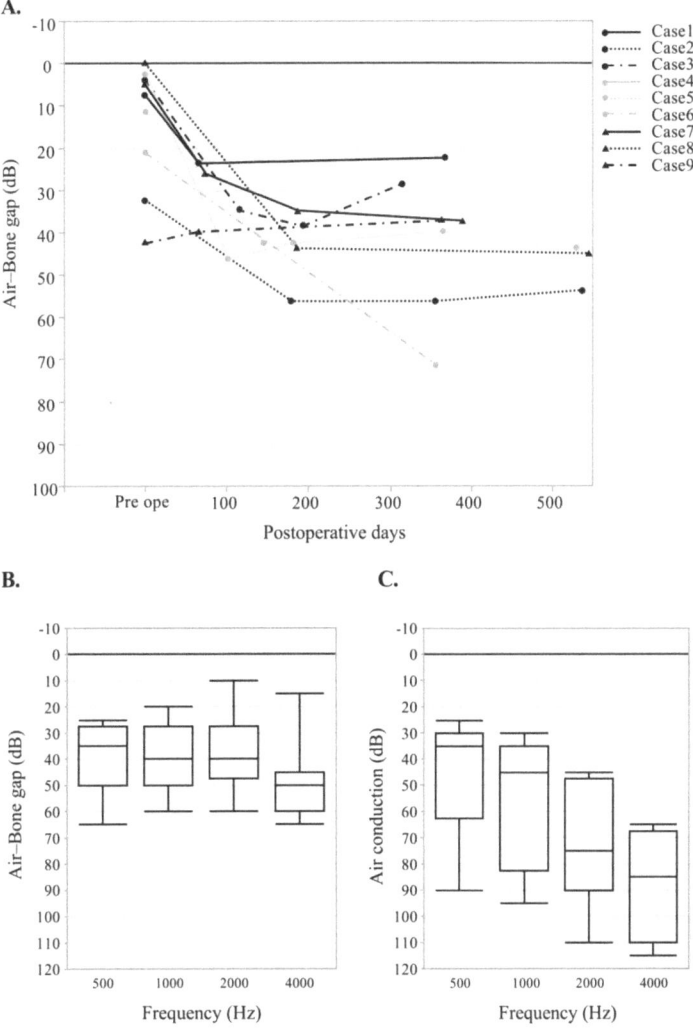

Figure 2. Postoperative hearing level of nine cases with reconstruction of the auditory canal with a free flap. (**A**) Hearing outcome of air–bone gap after surgery in nine patients. (**B**) Air–bone gap by frequency after surgery. (**C**) Air conduction level by frequency after surgery. The horizontal line within the box represents the median sample value. Box boundaries represent the 1st and 3rd quartiles. Whiskers extend from quartiles to the minimum/maximum data point.

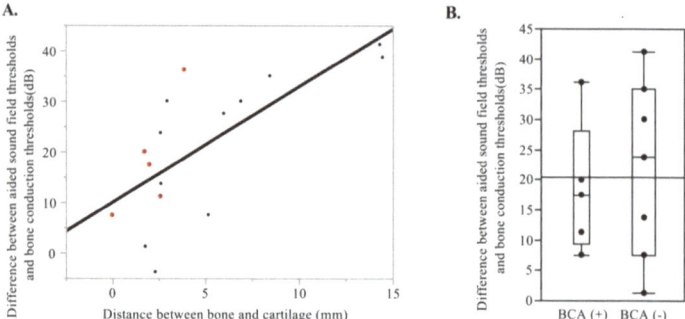

Figure 3. Effectiveness of the cartilage conduction hearing aid in cases after lateral temporal bone resection. (**A**) The relationship defining the distance between the auricular cartilage and the temporal bone and the difference between the aided sound field and bone conduction thresholds in 16 cases with the cartilage conduction hearing aids. Red dots show cases with BCA. (**B**) Difference between the aided sound field and bone conduction thresholds in 12 cases without external auditory meatus reconstruction. BCA; bone-cartilage anchoring.

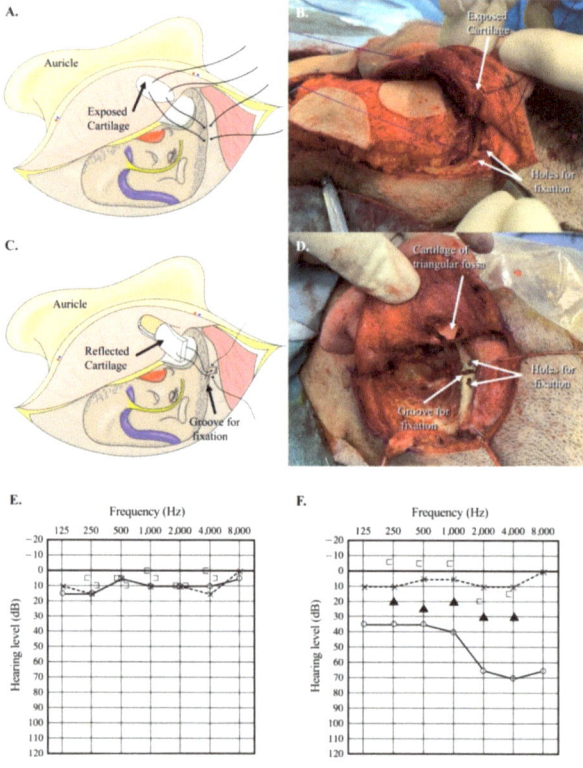

Figure 4. Bone–cartilage anchoring technique (BCA). (**A**) Auricular cartilage was anchored to the temporal bone with a 3-0 PDS suture (Type 1). (**B**) Surgical view of the Type 1 bone–cartilage anchoring technique (Case 13). (**C**) The auricular cartilage was inserted into the created groove of the temporal bone and fixed with a 3-0 PDS suture (Type 2). (**D**) Surgical view of the type 2 bone–cartilage anchoring technique (Case 12). (**E**) Preoperative pure-tone audiometry (Case 10). (**F**) Postoperative pure-tone audiometry of case 10 after the bone–cartilage anchoring technique. The black triangle shows the hearing level with a cartilage conduction hearing aid at a sound field with adequate masking on the contralateral side.

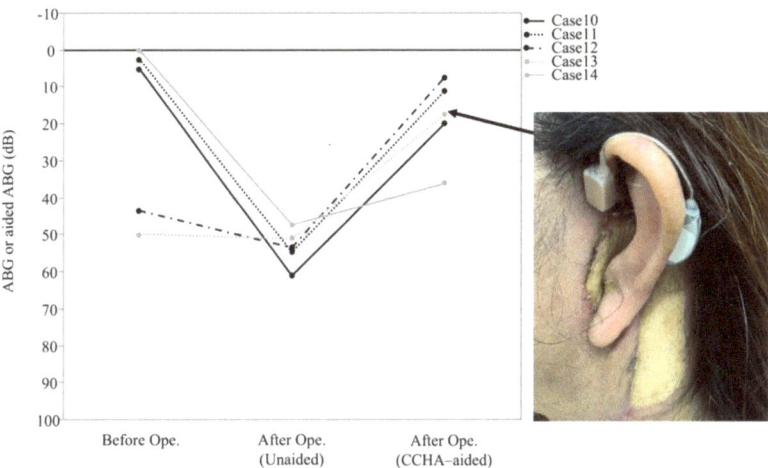

Figure 5. The outcome of the air–bone gap after the bone–cartilage anchoring technique surgery. An inset shows the auricular wearing the cartilage conduction hearing aid (Case 13). The CCHA transducer was fixed to the anterior root of the helix with double-sided tape. The difference between the aided sound field and bone conduction thresholds was represented as an air–bone gap under the CCHA-aided state after surgery. CCHA, cartilage conduction hearing aid; Ope., operation.

4. Discussion

The only currently considered standard of treatment for temporal bone malignancies in the world is en bloc and negative margin resection [11–13]. Previous reports have shown that patients with a negative margin resection have an excellent long-term prognosis in both early and advanced stages. LTBR and subtotal temporal bone resection (STBR) have been widely used for en bloc resection of temporal bone malignancies. STBR includes the resection of the inner ear structure, making it impossible to conserve hearing postoperatively. By contrast, LTBR preserves the inner ear structure, but this treatment will result in conductive hearing loss. Various reconstruction methods have been reported for postoperative temporal bone defects [14–17]. However, only a few reports have considered hearing preservation by combining tympanoplasty and external auditory canal reconstruction [3,4,18]. In 2016, the UK Guideline for Management of Lateral Skull Base Cancer was published. The guideline confirmed that a hearing deficit is an inevitable outcome of temporal bone resection but did not provide any reconstruction options to preserve hearing. The guideline did, however, describe rehabilitation for total hearing loss. Total conductive hearing loss can be rehabilitated through an osseointegrated bone-anchored hearing aid (BAHA) or a bilateral contralateral routing of signals aid [19].

Both complete resection of the tumor and hearing compensation after surgery are necessary to maintain the quality of life of patients. To date, there are four options to maintain or correct ipsilateral hearing: (1) reconstruction with a local flap, (2) reconstruction with a free pedicled flap, (3) middle ear implant or BAHA, and (4) bone conduction hearing aid. As of 1 April 2021, neither the middle ear implant or the BAHA for unilateral hearing deficit were covered by health insurance in Japan. Therefore, patients must choose from the other three options. Each option has advantages and disadvantages, as shown in Table 2.

In 2013, Iida et al. reported the reconstruction of the external auditory canal with a free flap after LTBR [18]. To reconstruct the external auditory canal, a relatively thin myocutaneous flap is needed. This limits the harvest site for a free flap to the forearm, groin, or anterolateral thigh. It is relatively easy to collect a flap thin enough to make the auditory canal from the forearm; however, because this is an exposed area, harvesting a flap may result in a cosmetic problem. A flap harvested from the groin can also be thin, but a long feeding blood vessel is difficult to collect in this area. The anterolateral thigh flap is thicker but has the advantage of being a less exposed area and having long feeding vessels, which convey a higher degree of freedom in anastomosis construction. In our institution, the anterolateral thigh flap is preferred for reconstruction (seven out of nine patients). When a tumor is considered resectable with negative surgical margins on preoperative CT and MRI scans, reconstruction of the external auditory canal with a free flap is considered if the patient wants to undergo hearing-preserving surgery. To avoid the risk of stenosis of the auditory canal, delayed wound healing, and complications from postoperative radiotherapy, a well-vascularized free flap is used for the reconstruction of the external auditory canal (if required) [20]. In our series, the subcutaneous tissue from the flap was removed to produce a thin layer of vascularized skin, which was used to reconstruct the tympanic membrane.

Table 2. Hearing compensation after temporal bone surgery.

Hearing Loss Compensation after Temporal Bone Resection	
Advantages	Disadvantages
Free Flap Reconstruction	
1. The possibility to maintain the hearing level without hearing aid	1. The postoperative volume of the flap can't be predicted preoperatively. Thusly, surgeon should explain the staged surgery to reduce the volume of the flap to maintain the external ear canal if necessary
2. The easy detection of the tumor recurrence through the canal	2. Need to clean the auditory canal regularly
3. The possibility to use the hearing aid with ear mold	3. The possibility of recurrent tumor exposure
	4. The ear mold is needed to be renewed depends on the volume of the flap
Local Flap Reconstruction	
1. Less invasive	1. Deterioration of the conductive hearing loss and otorrhea, caused by Stenosis, Contracture, chronic infection and bone exposure
2. The possibility to maintain the hearing level without hearing aid	2. Delay wound healing
3. The easy detection of the tumor recurrence through the canal	3. Dual local flaps and skin grafting are often needed
4. The possibility to use the hearing aid with ear mold	4. Need to clean the auditory canal regularly
Bone Conductive Haring Aid (No ear canal)	
1. No need of postoperative clean-up of the auditory canal	1. Strong contact to the skin and pressure against the cranial bone of bone-conductive hearing aid cause the skin erosion and patient's pain.
2. The maintain the hearing level with hearing aid	2. Residual and recurrent disease need to be detected only by radiological examination.
3. Prevent the tumor exposure when the tumor is recurrent	3. Expensive (purchasing expense, repair cost, etc.)
Cartilage Conductive Hearing (No ear canal)	
1. No need of postoperative clean-up of the auditory canal	1. Residual and recurrent disease need to be detected only by radiological examination.
2. Hearing aid is small and right	2. Expensive (purchasing expense, repair cost, etc.)
3. Prevent the tumor exposure when the tumor is recurrent	
4. No strong pressure to the skin and cranial bone	

It is well known that, in general, the volume of the free flap decreases gradually after surgery. However, not all cases involving free flap reconstruction follow the same clinical course. We encountered a case in which the volume of the free flap was conserved, resulting in stenosis of the reconstructed external auditory meatus (Case 6). Thus, the surgeon should preoperatively explain the possibility of a staged surgery to reduce the flap volume if necessary. Additionally, there is a possibility of deviation of the columella, resulting in worsening conductive hearing loss. Furthermore, hearing results depend on the patient. Only two patients achieved <30 dB of a mean postoperative ABG. Considering that hearing results largely rely on both patient factors and surgeon skills, there is a significant amount of room for improving this surgical procedure.

Adjuvant radiotherapy can cause osteoradionecrosis, the elevation of the sensorineural hearing thresholds, and radiation-induced otitis media and externa (dermatitis). Thus, LTBR with external auditory canal reconstruction and tympanoplasty is recommended only in cases with a high possibility of a margin-free resection based on the preoperative radiological evaluation. However, we cannot predict the result of a postoperative histopathological examination of all surgical cases. In our series, four out of nine patients had a positive margin resection, although the preoperative radiological assessment seemed to predict negative surgical margins. To prevent postoperative osteoradionecrosis of the temporal bone, the best option is to fill the surgical defect with well-vascularized tissue. Considering these aspects, an alternative method for postoperative hearing compensation is needed for cases with a high possibility of adjuvant radiotherapy.

Because a reconstructed auditory canal does not have a natural self-cleaning mechanism, cleaning the reconstructed auditory canal after surgery should also be considered. A preoperative explanation should be given to patients on how the reconstructed ear canal should be cleaned regularly for the rest of their life. On the other hand, strong contact with the skin and the pressure exerted against the cranial bone from the bone conduction hearing aids can cause skin erosion and pain. To overcome these disadvantages, we used a CCHA in a case with LTBR to maintain hearing postoperatively. In Japan, CCHAs have become commercially available [5–10]. This type of hearing aid is small and requires less pressure on the contact area. If the CCHA can compensate for postoperative hearing disturbances, the patient can avoid skin complications in the reconstructed ear canal. Furthermore, we considered that the desired hearing level could be achieved regardless of the surgical result of the reconstruction.

The hearing results of the patient with a CCHA after LTBR implied that the distance separating the auricular cartilage and the temporal bone is a potential factor for improving the effectiveness of sound transfer using the CCHAs after LTBR. With the cartilage anchored to the temporal bone, as shown in Figure 4, CCHAs may effectively transfer sound after LTBR. This technique is very simple, and every surgeon can provide the same quality of care. Results of the average difference between the aided sound field thresholds and bone conduction thresholds at 0.5, 1, 2 and 4 kHz in five cases with the cartilage conduction hearing devices are shown in Figure 5. We found a satisfactory result of less than 25 dB of mean postoperative difference between the aided sound field and bone conduction thresholds in four out of five cases (Figure 5).

Nishimura's group reported several advantages of CCHAs [5–10]. A CCHA includes both the cartilage–bone sound pathway and the cartilage air and direct air pathways. Furthermore, Morimoto et al. reported that fibrotic tissue connected to the ossicles provides an additional pathway, which is termed the fibrotic tissue pathway [21]. They mentioned that a substantial connection of occluding fibrotic tissue with the ossicles implied the presence of a fibrotic tissue pathway. We found a substantial connection of occluding fibrotic tissue with the ossicles in 10 out of 16 cases. These cases may use both the fibrotic tissue pathway and the cartilage–bone pathway. It has the advantage of aiding patients with outer ear disorders, such as atresia of the external auditory canal. This makes the approach suitable for cases that involve temporal bone resection. However, disconnection between the cartilage and bone may result in sound transmission disturbance. Our technique overcame this issue by compensating for hearing loss postoperatively with the CCHA. Furthermore, patients that use bone conduction hearing aids often suffer from pain and discomfort due to the strong contact that the aid has with the skin and the pressure that it exerts against the cranial bone. Cartilage conduction does not require strong and sustained pressure on the skin. Thus, we first introduced the CCHA in postoperative cases of LTBR. In these cases, the auditory canal was closed and they did not need to clean the auditory canal. Postoperative hearing in these cases was satisfactory. The bone–cartilage anchoring technique is a simple procedure to establish contact between the auricular cartilage and the temporal bone, which may improve sound transfer in patients with a CCHA after LTBR. It could be one effective option to compensate hearing ability after LTBR.

A limitation of this study was its small sample size. Further studies are warranted to validate our preliminary data. However, based on the present data, we predict that CCHAs will be introduced to more patients treated using the bone–cartilage anchoring technique.

5. Conclusions

This paper presented the hearing outcomes and options for hearing compensation after LTBR. The information obtained from our review can be extrapolated to offer guidance on reconstruction for these patients. Surgeons should consider hearing compensation for surgical cases of temporal bone malignancies as well as curative surgical resection.

Author Contributions: Conceptualization, N.K. and T.N. (Takashi Nakagawa); methodology, N.K.; validation, N.K., T.N. (Takashi Nakagawa); formal analysis, N.K. and S.M.; investigation, N.K.; resources, N.M., N.A.T. and T.N. (Teppei Noda); data curation, Y.H., K.I., T.T. and S.M.; writing—original draft preparation, N.K.; writing—review and editing, K.S., R.S., K.K., T.H., R.U., M.M. and R.K.; supervision, T.N. (Takashi Nakagawa); project administration, N.K. and T.N. (Takashi Nakagawa); funding acquisition, N.K. and T.N. (Takashi Nakagawa). All authors have read and agreed to the published version of the manuscript.

Funding: Part of this work was supported by the JSPS KAKENHI Grant (JP 18H02951 and 18K16895).

Institutional Review Board Statement: The study was conducted according to the guidelines of the Declaration of Helsinki, and approved by the ethics committee of Kyushu University Hospital (permit no. 29–43, approval date: 17 April 2017).

Informed Consent Statement: Informed consent was obtained from subjects or waived because of the retrospective nature of the study and the analysis used anonymous clinical data.

Data Availability Statement: The authors confirm that the data supporting the findings of this study are available within the article.

Conflicts of Interest: The authors report no personal financial support for this article and no conflicts of interest regarding any of the materials or devices described in this article.

References

1. Lovin, B.D.; Gidley, P.W. Squamous cell carcinoma of the temporal bone: A current review. *Laryngoscope Investig. Otolaryngol.* **2019**, *4*, 684–692. [CrossRef] [PubMed]
2. Moody, S.A.; Hirsch, B.E.; Myers, E.N. Squamous cell carcinoma of the external auditory canal: An evaluation of a staging system. *Am. J. Otol.* **2000**, *21*, 582–588. [PubMed]
3. Morita, S.; Nakamaru, Y.; Homma, A.; Sakashita, T.; Masuya, M.; Fukuda, S. Hearing preservation after lateral temporal bone resection for early-stage external auditory canal carcinoma. *Audiol. Neurootol.* **2014**, *19*, 351–357. [CrossRef] [PubMed]
4. Hoshikawa, H.; Miyashita, T.; Mori, N. Surgical procedures for external auditory canal carcinoma and the preservation of postoperative hearing. *Case Rep. Surg.* **2012**, *2012*, 841372. [CrossRef]
5. Hosoi, H.; Nishimura, T.; Shimokura, R.; Kitahara, T. Cartilage conduction as the third pathway for sound transmission. *Auris Nasus Larynx* **2019**, *46*, 151–159. [CrossRef]
6. Nishimura, T.; Hosoi, H.; Saito, O.; Miyamae, R.; Shimokura, R.; Matsui, T.; Iwakura, T. Benefit of a new hearing device utilizing cartilage conduction. *Auris Nasus Larynx* **2013**, *40*, 440–446. [CrossRef]
7. Nishimura, T.; Hosoi, H.; Saito, O.; Miyamae, R.; Shimokura, R.; Matsui, T.; Yamanaka, T.; Levitt, H. Is cartilage conduction classified into air or bone conduction? *Laryngoscope* **2014**, *124*, 1214–1219. [CrossRef]
8. Shimokura, R.; Hosoi, H.; Nishimura, T.; Yamanaka, T.; Levitt, H. Cartilage conduction hearing. *J. Acoust. Soc. Am.* **2014**, *135*, 1959–1966. [CrossRef]
9. Nishimura, T.; Hosoi, H.; Saito, O.; Miyamae, R.; Shimokura, R.; Yamanaka, T.; Kitahara, T.; Levitt, H. Cartilage conduction is characterized by vibrations of the cartilaginous portion of the ear canal. *PLoS ONE* **2015**, *10*, e0120135. [CrossRef]
10. Nishimura, T.; Hosoi, H.; Saito, O.; Shimokura, R.; Yamanaka, T.; Kitahara, T. Cartilage Conduction Hearing Aids for Severe Conduction Hearing Loss. *Otol. Neurotol.* **2018**, *39*, 65–72. [CrossRef]
11. Komune, N.; Noda, T.; Kogo, R.; Miyazaki, M.; Tsuchihashi, N.A.; Hongo, T.; Koike, K.; Sato, K.; Uchi, R.; Wakasaki, T.; et al. Primary Advanced Squamous Cell Carcinoma of the Temporal Bone: A Single-Center Clinical Study. *Laryngoscope* **2021**, *131*, E583–E589. [CrossRef]

12. Nakagawa, T.; Kumamoto, Y.; Natori, Y.; Shiratsuchi, H.; Toh, S.; Kakazu, Y.; Shibata, S.; Nakashima, T.; Komune, S. Squamous cell carcinoma of the external auditory canal and middle ear: An operation combined with preoperative chemoradiotherapy and a free surgical margin. *Otol. Neurotol.* **2006**, *27*, 242–248, discussion 249. [CrossRef]
13. Yin, M.; Ishikawa, K.; Honda, K.; Arakawa, T.; Harabuchi, Y.; Nagabashi, T.; Fukuda, S.; Taira, A.; Himi, T.; Nakamura, N.; et al. Analysis of 95 cases of squamous cell carcinoma of the external and middle ear. *Auris Nasus Larynx* **2006**, *33*, 251–257. [CrossRef]
14. Howard, B.E.; Nagel, T.H.; Barrs, D.M.; Donald, C.B.; Hayden, R.E. Reconstruction of Lateral Skull Base Defects: A Comparison of the Submental Flap to Free and Regional Flaps. *Otolaryngol. Head Neck Surg.* **2016**, *154*, 1014–1018. [CrossRef]
15. Moncrieff, M.D.; Hamilton, S.A.; Lamberty, G.H.; Malata, C.M.; Hardy, D.G.; Macfarlane, R.; Moffat, D.A. Reconstructive options after temporal bone resection for squamous cell carcinoma. *J. Plast. Reconstr. Aesthet. Surg.* **2007**, *60*, 607–614. [CrossRef]
16. Moore, M.G.; Lin, D.T.; Mikulec, A.A.; McKenna, M.J.; Varvares, M.A. The occipital flap for reconstruction after lateral temporal bone resection. *Arch. Otolaryngol. Head Neck Surg.* **2008**, *134*, 587–591. [CrossRef]
17. Resto, V.A.; McKenna, M.J.; Deschler, D.G. Pectoralis major flap in composite lateral skull base defect reconstruction. *Arch. Otolaryngol. Head Neck Surg.* **2007**, *133*, 490–494. [CrossRef]
18. Iida, T.; Mihara, M.; Yoshimatsu, H.; Narushima, M.; Koshima, I. Reconstruction of the external auditory canal using a super-thin superficial circumflex iliac perforator flap after tumour resection. *J. Plast. Reconstr. Aesthet. Surg.* **2013**, *66*, 430–433. [CrossRef]
19. Homer, J.J.; Lesser, T.; Moffat, D.; Slevin, N.; Price, R.; Blackburn, T. Management of lateral skull base cancer: United Kingdom National Multidisciplinary Guidelines. *J. Laryngol. Otol.* **2016**, *130*, S119–S124. [CrossRef]
20. Patel, N.S.; Modest, M.C.; Brobst, T.D.; Carlson, M.L.; Price, D.L.; Moore, E.J.; Janus, J.R. Surgical management of lateral skull base defects. *Laryngoscope* **2016**, *126*, 1911–1917. [CrossRef]
21. Morimoto, C.; Nishimura, T.; Hosoi, H.; Saito, O.; Fukuda, F.; Shimokura, R.; Yamanaka, T. Sound transmission by cartilage conduction in ear with fibrotic aural atresia. *J. Rehabil. Res. Dev.* **2014**, *51*, 325–332. [CrossRef] [PubMed]

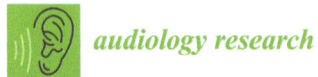

Review

How Is the Cochlea Activated in Response to Soft Tissue Auditory Stimulation in the Occluded Ear?

Miriam Geal-Dor [1,2] and Haim Sohmer [3,*]

1. Speech & Hearing Center, Hebrew University-Hadassah Medical School, Jerusalem 91200, Israel; gmiriam@hadassah.org.il
2. Department of Communication Disorders, Hadassah Academic College, Jerusalem 91200, Israel
3. Department of Medical Neurobiology (Physiology), Hebrew University-Hadassah Medical School, P.O. Box 12272, Jerusalem 91120, Israel
* Correspondence: haims@ekmd.huji.ac.il

Abstract: Soft tissue conduction is an additional mode of auditory stimulation which can be initiated either by applying an external vibrator to skin sites not overlying skull bone such as the neck (so it is not bone conduction) or by intrinsic body vibrations resulting, for example, from the heartbeat and vocalization. The soft tissue vibrations thereby induced are conducted by the soft tissues to all parts of the body, including the walls of the external auditory canal. In order for soft tissue conduction to elicit hearing, the soft tissue vibrations which are induced must penetrate into the cochlea in order to excite the inner ear hair cells and auditory nerve fibers. This final stage can be achieved either by an osseous bone conduction mechanism, or, more likely, by the occlusion effect: the vibrations of the walls of the occluded canal induce air pressures in the canal which drive the tympanic membrane and middle ear ossicles and activate the inner ear, acting by means of a more air conduction-like mechanism. In fact, when the clinician applies his stethoscope to the body surface of his patient in order to detect heart sounds or pulmonary air flow, he is detecting soft tissue vibrations.

Keywords: bone conduction; soft tissue conduction; occlusion effect; external canal; air conduction; vibrations; stethoscope

1. Introduction

An auditory sensation can be initiated by several modes of auditory stimulation, each of which activates the hair cells and auditory nerve fibers of the inner ear.

1.1. Air Conduction

In most situations, hearing is elicited by alternating condensation rarefaction air pressures, initiated by the vibrations of the sound producing structure. The vibrations are conducted to the ear by air (hence called air conduction—AC). In the inner ear, the AC sound gives rise to an apparent mechanical wave progressing along the basilar membrane, which has been called the traveling wave.

1.2. Bone Conduction

(BC) is an additional mode of auditory stimulation induced when a clinical bone vibrator is applied to skin sites overlying skull bone such as at the mastoid or forehead, and initiates vibrations of skull bone. It is used mainly in the clinic in order to differentiate between a conductive hearing loss (CHL) (in which AC thresholds are elevated, but BC thresholds are in the normal range) and a sensorineural hearing loss (SNHL) (in which both AC and BC thresholds are elevated). The bone vibrations are conducted along skull bone to the outer, middle and inner ears (therefore, called bone conduction, a definition based on the medium through which the vibrations are conducted to the ear), where they give rise to the four generally accepted mechanisms of bone conduction acting simultaneously in parallel: the occlusion effect of the outer ear, inertia of the middle ear ossicles, inner ear fluid inertia and inner ear distortion (compression and expansion) [1]. These parallel BC mechanisms are thought to elicit hearing by eventually inducing a traveling wave along the basilar membrane, as in AC hearing [1]. BC is also used as an alternative form of hearing aid (bone anchored hearing aid—BAHA) in patients who cannot use a conventional AC hearing aid, with discharging ears and congenital malformations of the external ear [2,3].

1.3. Soft Tissue Conduction

Hearing can also be elicited by the relatively recently understood mode called soft tissue conduction, in which vibrations are initiated in the soft tissues of the body. The vibrations are induced either by an external vibrator (e.g., the clinical bone vibrator applied to skin sites not overlying skull bone, so that it is distinct from BC) or occur naturally, intrinsically in the body, e.g., by vibrations resulting from the heartbeat or blood flow [4] or vibrations of the vocal cord during self-vocalization, as described by von Bekesy [5]. These vibrations are conducted by the soft tissues to all parts of the body, including to the ear (therefore called soft tissue conduction—STC), and somehow excite it [6,7]. When the external auditory canal is occluded, the intrinsic vibrations become audible [4,7]. An example of STC can be demonstrated to the reader by occluding their external auditory canal with their finger in order to reduce possible external masking sounds, while gently stroking the stubble on the cheek or an ear ring. The auditory sensation perceived in response to the gentle stroking is due to STC (it is distinct from AC, since the external canal was occluded; and not BC, since bone vibrations were not induced).

In the past, all forms of hearing which were not directly initiated by AC had been traditionally grouped together under the general term "bone conduction". However, given the present understanding of the nature of STC, it is now apparent that several auditory phenomena which had been originally referred to as being the result of BC, can now be shown to be elicited by STC: e.g., hearing one's own voice [5,8], hearing of maternal sounds by the fetus in utero [9], and pulsatile tinnitus [10]. Therefore, while hearing by BC is mainly used in the clinic in order to differentiate between a CHL and a SNHL by assessing and comparing thresholds to AC and BC, the term "osseous BC" should be applied to those modes of hearing which are based on induction of actual vibrations of skull bone, and lead to the vibration of the outer, middle and inner ears [1].

1.4. Final Stage

However, the final stage of the hearing which is initiated by STC has yet to be demonstrated. In order for the soft tissue vibrations induced either by the external bone vibrator or intrinsically, e.g., by the heartbeat, to elicit an auditory sensation (hearing), the vibrations of the soft tissues must penetrate into the cochlea and excite the inner ear hair cells and the auditory nerve fibers. This final stage has been the source of several conflicting studies. Is the final stage of STC (inner ear excitation) achieved by inducing vibrations of actual skull bone, as in osseous BC, involving initiation of a traveling wave along the basilar membrane [11] (i.e., an osseous mechanism), or by an alternative non-osseous mechanism [6]? The answer to this question is important, since knowledge of the mechanism could contribute to improvements in the diagnosis of hearing loss assessed by the determination of the thresholds to AC and BC stimulation, and in the development of better forms of bone hearing aids.

2. Soft Tissue Conduction

The purpose of the present review is, therefore, to evaluate several alternative mechanisms which have been suggested to serve as the final stage of hearing initiated by STC, i.e., how the inner ear is excited in response to STC stimulation; and how the vibrations of the soft tissues, which result from the delivery of a vibratory stimulus to sites on the skin (not overlying skull bone) or initiated intrinsically in the body (for example, by contractions of the heart), reach and excite the inner ear.

2.1. Acoustic Impedance

Can the low magnitude soft tissue vibrations induced by threshold intensity STC stimulation give rise to skull bone vibrations? In other words: can, for example, the gentle stroking of the stubble on the cheek or the intrinsic sounds coming from the heartbeat or blood flow [4] eventually induce vibrations of the more rigid dense skull bone? This question can be expressed in physical terms by considering the acoustic impedances (defined as the product of the density of the medium and the velocity of sound in that medium) of the conducting media involved. The acoustic impedance of bone is 7.8×10^6 kg/m^2 s; of typical soft tissues is 1.6×10^6 kg/m^2 s; of water is 1.48×10^6 kg/m^2 s; and of air is 0.0004×10^6 kg/m^2 s [12–14]. When the acoustic impedances of two contiguous media are similar, the vibrations in one media are efficiently conducted to the other. However, when they differ (described as an impedance mismatch), the vibrations are attenuated at the interface. For example, at an air–water interface, an AC sound would be attenuated by about 30 dB, and not penetrate into the water [14]. In this case, the middle ear serves as an impedance matching device [12]. Given the differences in acoustic impedance between soft tissue and bone, the vibrations of the soft tissues would theoretically be attenuated by about 70% (equivalent to about 7 dB) at the soft tissue–bone interface [13]. This attenuation can be overcome by elevating the magnitude of the vibrations of the soft tissues, for example, by increasing the intensity of the stimulus acting on the soft tissues.

This theoretical degree of attenuation has been confirmed in studies conducted in the course of the development of BAHAs: the thresholds of BAHA patients to the more conventional application of the bone vibrator to the skin over the bone were compared to the thresholds of the same patients to the delivery of the vibratory stimuli directly to the bone BAHA titanium implant after it had been integrated into the bone. The two stimulation sites were 2 cm apart. The thresholds to the stimulus delivered directly to the implant were about 10 dB lower (better) than those delivered at the nearby skin [2]. In a complementary experiment, the magnitudes of the acceleration levels at hearing threshold in response to the delivery of the vibratory stimulus to the skin were measured on the titanium implant, and were compared to those measured on the nearby intact skin. The acceleration levels were about 20 dB lower (better) at threshold when measured directly on the implant [3]. In other words, the intensity of the vibratory stimuli delivered to the skin would have had to be about 10 dB greater than those delivered directly to the bone (i.e., the implant) in order to enable the stimulus to the skin overlying the bone to reach threshold and (apparently) induce vibrations of the underlying bone.

2.2. Is Bone Conduction the Final Stage?

A recent study [11] made use of the titanium implant integrated in the mastoid bone of five BAHA patients in order to measure the magnitude of the skull vibrations on the implant in response to several intensities of vibratory stimulation delivered to a soft tissue site (neck), which represents STC. In the same patients, behavioral thresholds were also assessed to the same stimuli applied at the neck site. The amplitudes of the bone vibrations were found to be linearly related to the STC (neck) stimulus intensities. However, the authors were unable to detect vibrations at actual behavioral threshold due to the inherent background noise accompanying body activity in live human patients (e.g., respiration, circulation, movements). The lowest intensity at which vibrations could be detected in response to stimulation at the neck in all five of the participants was 50 dB HL, and vibrations could be detected in three of the five participants at 30 dB HL. The vibration magnitudes measured on the implant in response to higher intensity stimuli were therefore linearly extrapolated by the authors down to the intensity which had been the behavioral threshold of the same participants, in order to obtain an estimate of the magnitude of the vibrations at threshold. The authors concluded from the linearity that STC (neck) thresholds were directly elicited by bone vibrations, i.e., by an osseous mechanism. However, this cannot be taken as evidence that the final stage of STC is osseous, since, though linearly related to the intensity of the STC stimulation at the neck, at some low level of the vibrations of the soft tissue, the magnitude of these vibrations would be below threshold; a non-osseous mechanism cannot be excluded; and the linear extrapolation may not provide the magnitude of the vibrations at actual threshold. Furthermore, as described above, the vibratory stimuli delivered to the skin overlying the mastoid bone would have to be about 10 dB greater in intensity in order to reach the threshold by an osseous mechanism. Therefore, all the more so, the vibrations within the soft tissues which had been elicited in response to threshold-level stimuli delivered to the neck STC site would surely not be able to induce vibrations of the mastoid bone, and a non-osseous mechanism is likely involved. It has been suggested that this is due to the soft tissues acting as a "shunt" for the vibratory stimuli [3], i.e., part of the vibratory energy was "dispersed" in the soft tissues, and not transmitted to the bone (as a result of the impedance mismatch). Also, since the attenuation of the STC-induced soft tissue vibrations at the soft tissue–bone interface is of the order of only 7 dB, the transition from a non-osseous mechanism which is effective at actual threshold to an osseous mechanism at some supra-threshold intensity may be undetectable when using 5 dB intensity steps.

Furthermore, in several examples of STC, additional evidence can be presented which suggests that the final stage of hearing may not involve an osseous mechanism. For instance, the fetus in utero, after about 20 weeks gestation, responds to maternal sounds. While these signs of fetal hearing have been ascribed to BC [9,15], it is now clear that the maternal sounds reach the fetus through the maternal and fetal soft tissues by STC [16]. However, the presence of amniotic fluid filling the fetal middle ear cavity [17], converts the impedance of the oval and round windows more similar to each other. Therefore, fetal hearing probably does not involve the BC mechanisms of inner ear fluid inertia and inner ear distortion, which are based on differences in the impedances between the two windows. In other words, the major osseous BC mechanisms effective in the adult ear [1], are greatly reduced in the fetal ear [18]. Furthermore, fetal skull bone is not fully developed, and there are membranous sutures between the component skull bones; hence, it likely would not be able to conduct vibrations directly along skull bone by bone conduction to the ear [19].

2.3. Occlusion Effect

In addition, in studies designed to elucidate the mechanisms of STC hearing [7,20–22], the external auditory canal of the participants was usually occluded with an ear plug in order to exclude the possibility that the participant would respond to the AC sounds accompanying the STC stimulus delivered by a bone vibrator, and in order to reduce external masking sounds. However, in the presence of the occluding ear plugs, the occlusion effect (OE) would likely be elicited. It has been shown that the OE results from vibrations of the walls of the external auditory canal [23,24] which are induced by the vibrations of the soft tissues initiated by the external bone vibrator, or by the intrinsic body sounds resulting, for example, from the heartbeat. In fact, when the clinician uses a stethoscope to detect these intrinsic body sounds (e.g., heartbeat, pulmonary air flow) in their physical examination of a patient, they are making use of the intrinsic vibrations, and this serves as a clear and obvious confirmation of the existence of soft tissue vibrations and soft tissue conduction [7]. Since soft tissue (skin) provides the immediate lining of the cavity of the canal including both the cartilaginous and the bony parts of the canal, it is likely that the OE is the result of the vibrations of the more compliant soft tissue-cartilaginous walls of the canal [7]. These vibrations produce air pressures in the occluded cavity which drive the tympanic membrane and the middle ear ossicles, and excite the inner ear by a mechanism similar to that in response to AC stimulation [7]. Furthermore, the hearing of self-vocalizations [5,8] and of one's own heartbeat and blood flow [4] when the external canal is occluded is also a result of the OE, in which the vibrations of the vocal cords during vocalization or the vibrations of the heart and blood flow are conducted by the soft tissues to the walls of the external auditory canal, leading to its vibration. It has also been shown that the OE elicited in response to the low frequency vibrations induced by the heartbeat and resulting blood flow reaches a magnitude of 40 to 50 dB [4], i.e., the sound pressure in the occluded external canal is 100 times greater than that in the open canal; and this would require relatively large excursions of an extensive area of the canal wall, probably the more compliant soft tissue-cartilaginous wall. The air pressures induced in the occluded canal drive the tympanic membrane and the middle ear ossicles, in a pathway similar to that in AC hearing [7] (see Figure 1). In addition, in the studies conducted on BAHA participants [11,25], the external auditory canal in the tested ear was occluded with an ear plug. Therefore, the OE was likely elicited, enhancing the sensitivity (reducing the threshold) of the BAHA participant. Thus, the STC vibrations induced by the bone vibrator at the neck STC site were conducted by means of STC to the external canal walls, causing their vibration. In the presence of the occluding ear plug, the sound pressure in the occluded ear canal would be elevated, driving the tympanic membrane, middle ear ossicles, exciting the inner ear by a mechanism based on a sequence of events similar to an AC pathway, i.e., leading to a traveling wave. Thus, while the OE is considered one of the component mechanisms of BC [1], the OE is likely the result of the vibrations of the soft tissue-cartilaginous part of the canal wall [7], and not of the bony part. This may also be the mechanism leading to hearing in response to the delivery of vibratory stimuli to fluid applied to the external canal (which is also a form of STC), which was effective mainly to the lower frequencies [26].

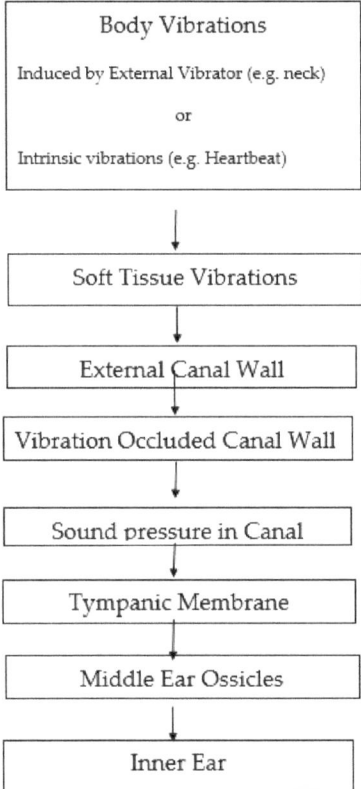

Figure 1. Schematic diagram showing the suggested mechanism of the final stage of hearing in response to soft tissue conduction: the vibrations of the soft tissues (initiated either by an external vibrator, for example, at the neck or by intrinsic body vibrations, e.g., heartbeat) elicit the occlusion effect, which produces sound pressure in the occluded external canal, and drive the tympanic membrane and the ossicular chain. Therefore, the inner ear is excited by a pathway similar to that in response to AC stimulation.

3. Conclusions

In conclusion, the OE enables the vibrations of the soft tissues to penetrate into the cochlea by means of the sound pressures in the occluded canal, and likely contributes a major component to the final stage of hearing in response to threshold intensity STC auditory stimulation.

Author Contributions: Conceptualization, H.S.; writing—original draft preparation, H.S.; writing—review and editing, M.G.-D. All authors have read and agreed to the published version of the manuscript.

Funding: The participation of M. Geal-Dor was supported by the Newman Fund for Audiological Research.

Institutional Review Board Statement: Not applicable.

Informed Consent Statement: Not applicable.

Data Availability Statement: Not applicable.

Conflicts of Interest: The authors declare no conflict of interest.

References

1. Stenfelt, S.; Goode, R.L. Bone-conducted sound: Physiological and clinical aspects. *Otol. Neurotol.* **2005**, *26*, 1245–1261. [CrossRef]
2. Håkansson, B.; Tjellström, A.; Rosenhall, U. Hearing thresholds with direct bone conduction versus conventional bone conduction. *Scand. Audiol.* **1984**, *13*, 3–13. [CrossRef]
3. Hakansson, B.; Tjellstrom, A.; Rosenhall, U. Acceleration levels at hearing threshold with direct bone conduction versus conventional bone conduction. *Acta Oto-Laryngol.* **1985**, *100*, 240–252. [CrossRef]
4. Stone, M.A.; Paul, A.M.; Axon, P.; Moore, B.C.J. A technique for estimating the occlusion effect for frequencies below 125 Hz. *Ear Hear.* **2014**, *35*, 49–55. [CrossRef]
5. Von Bekesy, G. The structure of the middle ear and the hearing of one's own voice by bone conduction. *J. Acoust. Soc. Am.* **1949**, *21*, 217–232. [CrossRef]
6. Sohmer, H. Soft tissue conduction: Review, mechanisms, and implications. *Trends Hear.* **2017**, *21*, 1–8. [CrossRef]
7. Geal-Dor, M.; Adelman, C.; Chordekar, S.; Sohmer, H. Occlusion Effect in Response to Stimulation by Soft Tissue Conduction-Implications. *Audiol. Res.* **2020**, *10*, 69–76. [CrossRef]
8. Reinfeldt, S.; Ostli, P.; Håkansson, B.; Stenfelt, S. Hearing one's own voice during phoneme vocalization–transmission by air and bone conduction. *J. Acoust. Soc. Am.* **2010**, *128*, 751–762. [CrossRef]
9. Sohmer, H.; Perez, R.; Sichel, J.Y.; Priner, R.; Freeman, S. The pathway enabling external sounds to reach and excite the fetal inner ear. *Audiol. Neurootol.* **2001**, *6*, 109–116. [CrossRef]
10. De Ridder, D.; Vanneste, S.; Menovsky, T. Pulsatile tinnitus due to a tortuous siphon-like internal carotid artery successfully treated by arterial remodeling. *Case Rep. Otolaryngol.* **2013**, *2013*, 938787. [CrossRef]
11. Chordekar, S.; Perez, R.; Adelman, C.; Sohmer, H.; Kishon-Rabin, L. Does hearing in response to soft-tissue stimulation involve skull vibrations? A within-subject comparison between skull vibration magnitudes and hearing thresholds. *Hear. Res.* **2018**, *364*, 59–67. [CrossRef] [PubMed]
12. Wever, E.G.; Lawrence, M. The function of the middle ear. In *Physiological Acoustics*; Princeton University Press: Princeton, NJ, USA, 1954; pp. 69–78.
13. Baun, J. Interaction with soft tissue. In *Physical Principles of General and Vascular Sonography*; ProSono Publishing: San Francisco, CA, USA, 2004; pp. 28–41.
14. Blakley, B.W.; Siddique, S. A qualitative explanation of the Weber test. *Otolaryngol. Head Neck Surg.* **1999**, *120*, 1–4. [CrossRef]
15. Gerhardt, K.J.; Huang, X.; Arrington, K.E.; Meixner, K.; Abrams, R.M.; Antonelli, P.J. Fetal sheep in utero hear through bone conduction. *Am. J. Otolaryngol.* **1996**, *17*, 374–379. [CrossRef]
16. Adelman, C.; Chordekar, S.; Perez, R.; Sohmer, H. Investigation of the mechanism of soft tissue conduction explains several perplexing auditory phenomena. *J. Basic Clin. Physiol. Pharmacol.* **2014**, *25*, 269–272. [CrossRef] [PubMed]
17. Priner, R.; Perez, R.; Freeman, S.; Sohmer, H. Mechanisms responsible for postnatal middle ear amniotic fluid clearance. *Hear. Res.* **2003**, *175*, 133–139. [CrossRef]
18. Karlsen, S.J.; Bull-Njaa, T.; Krokstad, A. Measurement of sound emission by endoscopic lithotripters: An in vitro study and theoretical estimation of risk of hearing loss in a fetus. *J. Endourol.* **2001**, *15*, 821–826. [CrossRef]
19. Opperman, L.A. Cranial sutures as intramembranous bone growth sites. *Dev. Dyn.* **2000**, *219*, 472–485. [CrossRef]
20. Ito, T.; Roosli, C.; Kim, C.J.; Sim, J.H.; Huber, A.M.; Probst, R. Bone conduction thresholds and skull vibration measured on the teeth during stimulation at different sites on the human head. *Audiol. Neurootol.* **2011**, *16*, 12–22. [CrossRef]
21. Watanabe, T.; Bertoli, S.; Probst, R. Transmission pathways of vibratory stimulation as measured by subjective thresholds and distortion-product otoacoustic emissions. *Ear Hear.* **2008**, *29*, 667–673. [CrossRef]
22. Geal-Dor, M.; Chordekar, S.; Adelman, C.; Sohmer, H. Bone conduction thresholds without bone vibrator application force. *J. Am. Acad. Audiol.* **2015**, *26*, 645–651. [CrossRef]

23. Fagelson, M.A.; Martin, F.N. The occlusion effect and ear canal sound pressure level. *Am. J. Audiol.* **1998**, *7*, 50–54. [CrossRef]
24. Goldstein, D.P.; Hayes, C.S. The occlusion effect in bone conduction hearing. *J. Speech Hear. Res.* **1965**, *8*, 137–148. [CrossRef] [PubMed]
25. Chordekar, S.; Perez, R.; Adelman, C.; Sohmer, H.; Kishon-Rabin, L. The Effect of Soft Tissue Stimulation on Skull Vibrations and Hearing Thresholds in Humans. *Otol. Neurotol.* **2021**. Online ahead of print. [CrossRef] [PubMed]
26. Geal-Dor, M.; Chordekar, S.; Adelman, C.; Kaufmann-Yehezkely, M.; Sohmer, H. Audiogram in Response to Stimulation Delivered to Fluid Applied to the External Meatus. *J. Audiol. Otol.* **2020**, *24*, 79–84. [CrossRef]

MDPI AG
Grosspeteranlage 5
4052 Basel
Switzerland
Tel.: +41 61 683 77 34

Audiology Research Editorial Office
E-mail: audiolres@mdpi.com
www.mdpi.com/journal/audiolres

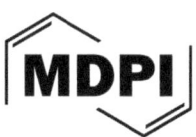

Disclaimer/Publisher's Note: The title and front matter of this reprint are at the discretion of the Guest Editor. The publisher is not responsible for their content or any associated concerns. The statements, opinions and data contained in all individual articles are solely those of the individual Editor and contributors and not of MDPI. MDPI disclaims responsibility for any injury to people or property resulting from any ideas, methods, instructions or products referred to in the content.

www.ingramcontent.com/pod-product-compliance
Lightning Source LLC
LaVergne TN
LVHW070002100526
83820ZLV00019B/2612